Praise for *The Parents' Guide to Clubfoot*

"Betsy Miller's *The Parents' Guide to Clubfoot* provides an excellent description of what the correction of clubfoot entails. It's incredibly useful to have all of this information, well organized, in one spot. As a parent of two sons born with severe clubfoot, I've definitely "been there." It is exciting to see that this first comprehensive parents' guide to clubfoot treatment focuses exclusively on the Ponseti method, because it is now the standard of care."

— Suzan, parent

"Betsy Miller has written an informative book specifically for parents that explains clubfoot in easy-to-understand terms. The book is quite in-depth and covers a wealth of information. In it you will learn about clubfoot, the process of treating clubfoot—from initial diagnosis to ongoing at-home treatment—and even how to help your child cope with the diagnosis. What I like about Betsy's book is that she is extraordinarily thorough. Knowing all current medical and treatment information removes the specter of second-guessing. Betsy talks about treatment for babies, treatment for older children, sleeping issues, coping with braces, and more. She also inserts individual success stories to make the book more personal. This guide is a valuable tool for any parent who has a baby or child with clubfoot."

— Nancy Konigsberg, MA, OTR/L

Ordering
Trade bookstores in the U.S. and Canada please contact:

Publishers Group West
1700 Fourth Street, Berkeley CA 94710
Phone: (800) 788-3123   Fax: (800) 351-5073

Hunter House books are available at bulk discounts for textbook course adoptions;
to community, health-care, and government organizations; and
for special promotions and fund-raising. For details please contact:

Special Sales Department
Hunter House Inc., PO Box 2914, Alameda CA 94501-0914
Phone: (510) 865-5282   Fax: (510) 865-4295
E-mail: ordering@hunterhouse.com

Individuals can order our books from most bookstores,
by calling **(800) 266-5592**, or from our website at
www.hunterhouse.com

THE PARENTS' GUIDE

to

CLUBFOOT

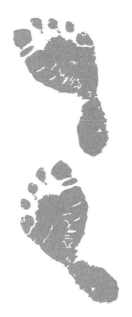

BETSY MILLER

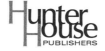

Hunter House PUBLISHERS

Hunter House Inc., Publishers
PO Box 2914
Alameda CA 94501-0914

Library of Congress Cataloging-in-Publication Data
Miller, Betsy, 1961-
The parents' guide to clubfoot / Betsy Miller.
   p. cm.
Includes bibliographical references and index.
ISBN 978-0-89793-614-9 (pbk.)
1. Clubfoot — Popular works. 2. Foot — Diseases — Popular works. 3. Foot — Abnormalities — Popular works. 4. Clubfoot — Treatment — Popular works.
I. Title.
RD783.M55 2012
617.5'8506 — dc23   2011037491

Project Credits

Cover Design: Brian Dittmar Design, Inc.
Book Production: John McKercher
Illustrations: Loney Grabscheid and Kelly Carter
Copy Editor: Amy Bauman
Proofreader: Lori Cavanaugh
Indexer: Candace Hyatt
Managing Editor: Alexandra Mummery
Publisher: Kiran S. Rana

Acquisitions Assistant: Elana Fiske
Publicity Assistant: Winona Azure
Rights Coordinator: Candace Groskreutz
Customer Service Manager: Christina Sverdrup
Order Fulfillment: Washul Lakdhon
Administrator: Theresa Nelson
Computer Support: Peter Eichelberger

Printed and bound by Sheridan Books, Ann Arbor, Michigan
Manufactured in the United States of America

9 8 7 6 5 4 3 2 1   First Edition   12 13 14 15 16

Contents

Important Note

The material in this book is intended to provide a review of information regarding clubfoot, also called talipes or congenital talipes equinovarus (CTEV). Every effort has been made to provide accurate and dependable information. The contents of this book have been compiled through professional research and in consultation with medical and mental-health professionals. However, health-care professionals have differing opinions, and advances in medical and scientific research are made very quickly, so some of the information may become outdated.

Therefore, the publisher, authors, and editors, as well as the professionals quoted in the book, cannot be held responsible for any error, omission, or dated material. The content of this book is for informational purposes; it is not a substitute for professional medical advice. Consult a physician about any medical symptoms or conditions that you or your child may have. Any use of the information in this book is at the reader's discretion. The author and the publisher specifically disclaim any and all liability arising directly or indirectly from the use or application of any information contained in this book in a program of self-care or under the care of a licensed practitioner.

Brand and product names commonly are trademarks or registered trademarks of their respective holders. Readers should contact the appropriate companies for more complete information regarding trademarks and registration.

Acknowledgments

I would like to thank my husband, Tom, and daughters, Katie and Tessa, for their understanding, support, and unfailing encouragement while I was writing this book.

Thank you to Michael Colburn, DPM, Matthew Dobbs, MD, and Jose Morcuende, MD, for allowing me to draw on their extensive experience and medical expertise in clubfoot treatment. Rebecca Bennett, RNMS/PNP/FNP-BC, has been a terrific resource in pain management. Thanks also to Jon Wilson, OSP, at Hanger Orthopedic Group; Suzan Carmichael, PhD; and Jean Colburn, RN, CDE.

Laura Geele Wang, Dr. Anthony Francis, and Patricia Zylius provided invaluable editorial assistance. Judi Brown, Susan Mittman, Elaine Lahey, Jerry Lahey, Sara Lahey, Ily Mason, Marcia Matthews, and Donna Tapella provided suggestions and support, which were greatly appreciated.

Many thanks to the members of the nosurgery4clubfoot online group, for practical comments and suggestions about the content of this book. Contributions from parents (and their children) in the trenches added so much to the book. Thank you to Asher Allen: David Allen: Isaac Allen: Jasper Avtarovski; Suzan Carmichael; Farley Dugan; Nicki Dugan; Katerina Haviara; Pamela Karydas; Keiran Korver; Lori Jo Learned-Burton, MD; Jocelyn Mace; Amy Rohr; Tamesin Salehian; Kristin Trangsrud; Jennifer Trevillian; Kimberly Wells; Tovey Wonnenberg; and all the other parents out there who provide each other with practical advice and emotional support in caring for children with clubfoot.

1
Understanding Clubfoot

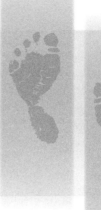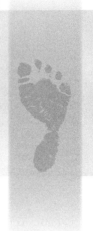

Clubfoot, also called talipes equinovarus (TEV) or congenital talipes equinovarus (CTEV), is a disorder that affects the foot and calf muscles. The foot tilts sideways and turns inward, and the heel is up high. The foot stays in this position unless it is treated. The calf muscles have fewer muscle fibers than usual, resulting in a thinner, higher calf. Clubfoot develops before a baby is born and can sometimes be seen in ultrasound during the mother's pregnancy. It can occur in both feet or in only one foot.

Clubfoot is treated as early as possible, usually within two weeks after birth. The goal of treatment is a foot that works well, is pain free, and looks normal. The most common clubfoot treatment in the United States is the Ponseti method. With this method, the doctor corrects the foot with stretching and casts, after which the child wears a brace. This method is endorsed by the Pediatric Orthopedic Society of North America (POSNA), the American Academy of Orthopedic Surgeons (AAOS), the European Paediatric Orthopaedic Society (EPOS), and many other medical organizations worldwide. Children and adults whose clubfeet were corrected with the Ponseti method typically do very well in the long term. Pamela has this to say about her son Dino, whose clubfeet were treated with the Ponseti method:

> Dino is now nine years old, his corrected feet are just perfect, and yesterday he figured out windsurfing. He's got his green belt in karate, is learning to play tennis, and is looking forward to another winter of snowboarding. My years-ago fears about his having underdeveloped calf muscles came to nothing; his little legs are quite muscular and very strong.   [PAMELA]

The photos in Figure 1.1 show a baby's feet before and after correction.

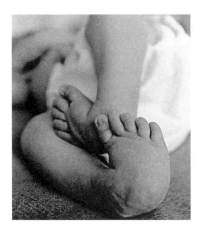
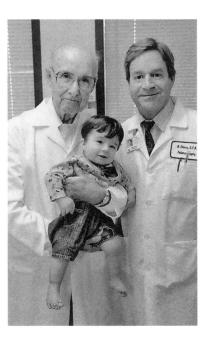

FIGURE 1.1. Isaac's feet before and after correction. The late Dr. Ignacio Ponseti, here with Dr. Michael Colburn, is holding Isaac. *(Photos courtesy of David Allen.)*

For about 50 percent of babies with clubfeet, both feet are affected. These babies have bilateral clubfoot. Babies who have only one clubfoot have unilateral clubfoot. Sometimes the foot is called a left clubfoot (LCF; see Figure 1.2) or right clubfoot (RCF).

If you look at a clubfoot from the outside, it might seem simple to move the foot into a normal position. This is not the case. Correcting the foot is complicated because there are many bones, tendons, and ligaments that work together to move the foot.

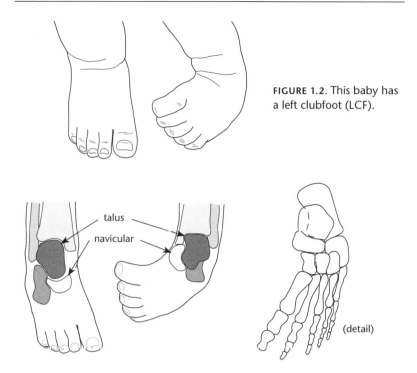

FIGURE 1.2. This baby has a left clubfoot (LCF).

talus

navicular

(detail)

FIGURE 1.3. A normal foot and clubfoot bone structure

The bones most affected by clubfoot are the tarsal bones, located in the middle of the foot. Some of these are in the wrong position, and in some babies they are also the wrong shape. Figure 1.3 shows how the bones in the foot are aligned for a normal foot and a clubfoot.

With clubfoot, many small bones in the middle of the foot (tarsal bones) are in the wrong position. Each tarsal bone has its own name, such as the talus and the navicular. Normally, the heel bone (calcaneus) is below the talus bone. In clubfoot, it is out of alignment and closer to the instep than usual.

Clubfoot affects the tendons and ligaments in the foot and calf, as well as the calf muscle. The foot tendons and ligaments located toward the instep and in the heel are shorter than usual. The tendons and ligaments on the other side of the foot (opposite the arch) are stretched out. Though each foot is unique, clubfoot problems can be grouped into these main areas:

- **Equinus.** The heel stays up and cannot move down.
- **Varus.** The foot is turned inward toward the midline of the body.
- **Supination.** This is a movement in the middle of the foot. To feel the movement that occurs with clubfoot, stand barefoot on the floor and shift your weight to the outside of your feet. Your big toes might come up off the floor when you do this.
- **Adductus.** The front of the foot turns in. Sometimes the foot looks like it is curved into a "C" shape.
- **Cavus.** The arch of the foot is too high.

Some cases of complex clubfoot also include a big toe that sticks up (is hyperextended), a crease on the sole of the foot, or a crease where the heel meets the ankle.

Types of Clubfoot

Clubfoot can be typical or atypical, and in rare cases it is associated with a syndrome. A syndrome is a group of symptoms or problems that occur together.

- **Typical clubfoot (also called idiopathic clubfoot).** This is the most common type of clubfoot. The cause is unknown, and the baby has no other problems that are related to the clubfoot.
- **Atypical clubfoot (also called complex clubfoot).** The clubfoot is more severe and should be treated by a doctor who is highly skilled in clubfoot treatment. The foot can be short and stubby. There is a crease on the sole of the foot, and in some cases there is also a crease at the top of the heel.
- **Clubfoot with a syndrome.** The doctor develops an individual treatment plan depending on the syndrome. Arthrogryposis (AMC), amniotic band syndrome (ABS), and meningomyelocele (also called spina bifida) are syndromes.

Untreated Clubfoot

A child who does not get treatment for clubfoot is unusual in the United States. This is more common in the developing world or in locations where treatment resources are limited. But even if treatment is delayed, the Ponseti method can be used to improve the child's foot before surgery is considered. The treatment protocol is different for these children.

If you can imagine trying to walk on the side of your foot, you will quickly realize some of the effects that would occur. The most common problems with untreated clubfoot are mobility limitations and chronic pain due to deformed bones and weight bearing on the wrong part of the feet. The shapes that a child's bones and joints grow into are affected by their alignment and how they are used. Over time, if the clubfoot is not corrected, the foot bones continue to grow into the wrong shapes, making clubfoot harder to correct. The knee and hip bones also become deformed due to the way the leg is rotated.

Why Clubfoot Occurs

In most cases, when clubfoot occurs, the reason is not known, though it does run in some families. Studies have reported the incidence of clubfoot as 1 in 800 or 1 in 1,000. It is more common in certain populations. Risk factors for clubfoot are listed here.

- **Unknown reasons.** In about 75 percent of cases, it is not known why clubfoot occurred. In these cases, there is no known family history of the condition, and it might not occur again within that family.

- **Family history.** About 25 percent of clubfoot cases occur in families in which another family member has clubfoot. Recently, researchers have discovered a gene associated with some cases of clubfoot.

- **Gender.** Clubfoot is twice as common in boys as in girls.

- **Syndromes.** Certain syndromes make it more likely that a child will have clubfoot. Some of these are arthrogryposis (AMC), amniotic band syndrome (ABS), and meningomyelocele (also called spina bifida). These conditions are rare. Most cases of clubfoot are not related to a syndrome.

It is only natural to ask why someone has a condition like clubfoot. Many parents wonder if they did something to cause it, or if they could have prevented it in some way. Though these risk factors make it more likely that a person will have clubfoot, it cannot be predicted or prevented. It isn't anyone's fault, but treatment can help your child. If you're worried about having another child with clubfoot, bear in mind that there is about a 96 percent chance that your next child will not have clubfoot.[1]

Physical Exam for Clubfoot

When a child is born with clubfoot, it is standard practice for the child to be referred to a specialist. Some clinics or hospitals have clubfoot centers. Usually the child is seen by a pediatric orthopedic doctor, though in some cases they are seen by a podiatrist. Though few podiatrists are trained in the Ponseti method, those who are can provide treatment just as effectively. Pediatric orthopedic doctors diagnose and treat bone and joint problems in babies and children. Podiatrists diagnose and treat foot problems for patients of all ages. The doctor does a physical exam, which typically includes the following:

- The doctor examines the child for any other problems in addition to the clubfoot that could affect the clubfoot treatment.
- The doctor checks the size and shape of the child's foot and calf. If only one foot is affected, the clubfoot is compared to the other foot.
- The child's foot is gently moved into different positions to measure its flexibility. The doctor feels the position of various foot bones as the foot moves to see which ones can move toward a better alignment.
- For a child who can walk, the doctor checks for patterns of calluses on the foot that show which part of the foot the child walks on.

The exam reveals whether the child has clubfoot or another condition that could resemble clubfoot, such as metatarsus adductus (MA). With MA, for example, a baby's foot is at an unusual angle but easily moves to a normal position; this is not the same as clubfoot.

[1] Children's Hospital Boston, "What Causes Clubfoot?" http://www.childrens hospital.org/az/Site1159/mainpageS1159P1.html (accessed 25 October 2011).

Usually the doctor does not need to take X rays to diagnose clubfoot. In cases where X rays are needed, a health-care worker such as a medical radiation technologist X rays the child's foot using a dose of radiation that is as low as possible. The X ray is targeted so that the X-ray beam exposes only the foot. It is best to go to an X-ray facility experienced in pediatrics with equipment calibrated for babies and children.

Doctors have different methods that they use to check how far out of alignment the foot is and whether it is flexible and can easily move toward a better alignment or is stiff and resistant. Many doctors use one of these methods:

- **Clubfoot Severity Scale (Diméglio Scale).** This is one of the most popular methods of assessing clubfoot. It is a scale from 0 to 20, with 0 indicating a normal foot and 20 indicating the most severe clubfoot.

- **Pirani Severity Score.** This method is also widely used. It takes into account six parts of the foot that can be affected by clubfoot. Each is scored as 0 (normal), 0.5 (moderate), or 1 (severe). Then the scores are added up.

- **Caroll Score.** The doctor checks for ten problems in the foot.

For more information, see "Clubfoot Assessment" on page 122.

Coping with Your Child's Diagnosis

Many parents of children born with clubfoot have similar reactions. Finding out your child has clubfoot can be a shock. When Nicki was pregnant with her second son, Farley, she found out during ultrasound that he had clubfoot. Here is how she describes her feelings:

I went to my twenty-week ultrasound with that usual euphoria over being able to "meet" my kid. I left devastated by the news that he had clubfoot. I feared the worst. I called my pediatrician on a Friday night and got no reassurances about a "normal" life. He said treatment consisted of castings and likely surgery, with stiffness, scar tissue, and arthritis to follow. His foot would never really be normal. Plenty of orthopedic surgeons could take care of this. His only silver lining was, "In the grand scheme of deformities, it could be a lot worse."

Through my tears, I hit the Internet and found the [nosurgery 4clubfoot] group. I studied photos of feet, casts, and bars. I read about pressure blisters and unqualified doctors whose work needed correction. I wrote to Dr. [Ignacio] Ponseti and asked [for a referral]. We had to drive forty-five minutes to see a doctor outside our network. It sounded overwhelming. But I talked to Dr. [Michael] Colburn before Farley was born, and he gave all the reassurances I'd been seeking. "Don't worry. Just enjoy your baby. Come see me when you're ready. It doesn't have to be minutes after he's born. He will be fine. We will fix this. Don't worry."

I detached myself from this pregnancy anyway. Could I love a kid with a deformity the way I loved my first? But when Farley arrived, I loved and studied that sweet little crooked foot. So tiny. So unique. He proved to be my little trooper. On day five, off to Dr. Colburn we drove. Farley fell asleep during his first casting. And his second…and third…and seven weeks later, nary a peep during his tenotomy. His foot came out beautiful, if just a little wrinkled at the ankle.   [NICKI]

Many times a baby's clubfoot is seen in an ultrasound during the mother's pregnancy. In most cases this is accurate, but sometimes when the baby is born it turns out that they do not have clubfoot after all. For example, the baby could have metatarsus adductus (MA), which can look similar to clubfoot but usually corrects itself without treatment. A recent study found a false-positive rate of 19 percent in prenatal clubfoot diagnoses.[2] A false-positive result means that the baby was thought to have clubfoot before birth but did not. The study found that false-positive results are more likely when the clubfoot

[2] Glotzbecker, M. P., et al., "Prenatally Diagnosed Clubfeet: Comparing Ultrasonographic Severity with Objective Clinical Outcomes," *Journal of Pediatric Orthopedics* 30, no. 6 (2010 Sep.): 606–11.

appears to be mild in the ultrasound, and the authors recommended developing more precise ways to assess clubfoot that is revealed in ultrasound.

A clubfoot diagnosis during pregnancy can be helpful because it gives you time to learn about clubfoot and to locate a doctor skilled in treating clubfoot. However, it also creates stress and anxiety. A health-care worker might ask you about terminating the pregnancy. The protocol for this varies depending on where you live. This is a sensitive issue that many people feel strongly about. Bear in mind that in most cases of clubfoot there is nothing else wrong with the baby. Having clubfoot does not mean that a baby has a syndrome (a group of symptoms or problems that occur together). However, babies with certain syndromes are at increased risk for clubfoot. If you think your baby might have a syndrome, ask a geneticist to explain what the syndrome is and whether there is a definite diagnosis.

Tovey's son Jack's clubfoot was successfully treated with the Ponseti method. She offers this advice to parents who are worried about their children's clubfoot:

It is normal to be anxious over your kids, especially kids with extra worries. I am a control freak but was blessed with the no-worries gene. My mom said the other day how fortunate that Jack was born to me and not her, because she would be a nervous wreck. That is not to say that I don't wonder what the future will hold, but I have faith that we have done the best for Jack's feet, and [we] take one day at a time. I think I was more worried in the beginning, too. Now at twenty months, Jack runs around like a maniac, and he has met all his little baby milestones early, so I can kind of relax. Don't stress. Just take it one step at a time.   [TOVEY]

Finding a doctor who is skilled in treating clubfoot and with whom you are comfortable is important. The next chapter gives more detail about a diagnosis of clubfoot and describes the recommended treatments.

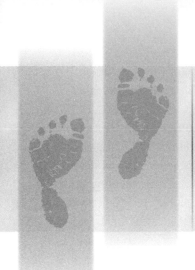

2

Preparing for Treatment

This chapter examines treatment for clubfoot, how doctors describe a clubfoot diagnosis, and medical conditions that can be associated with clubfoot. It also covers the role of doctors and healthcare workers and offers some basic advice about medical insurance and other types of financial support for treatment. The goal of treatment is for your child to have a foot that works well, is pain free, and looks normal, with as little surgery as possible.

In the past, doctors tried different ways to correct clubfoot. They found that forcing the foot into a normal position did not completely correct the clubfoot and could hurt the foot. Some types of surgery that were meant to correct clubfoot caused scarring that led to more foot problems as the child grew older. Today the most common clubfoot treatments are the Ponseti method and the French method of physical therapy. Because the Ponseti method is the main treatment in the United States, this book focuses on the Ponseti method. The French method requires ongoing, frequent visits with a physical therapist and extensive parent participation. It is not widely practiced in the United States, though the clubfoot center at Texas Scottish Rite Hospital for Children provides treatment with both the Ponseti method and the French physical therapy method. See "Infant Massage (Not Part of Treatment)" on page 96.

The Ponseti Method

The Ponseti method is a treatment for clubfoot that was developed by Dr. Ignacio Ponseti. One of the things that Dr. Ponseti discovered in his pioneering work with clubfoot treatment is that many bones in the foot can move in different directions, not just up and down or side to side. He also found that the sequence of adjustments matters, and, knowing this, he was able to recommend the most effective approach to correcting the foot. It is like solving a three-dimensional puzzle with pieces that can slide in different directions. Moving the wrong pieces might solve one part of the puzzle, but only if the pieces are moved in the right sequence, can the puzzle be completely solved.

Today the Ponseti method is endorsed by the Pediatric Orthopedic Society of North America (POSNA), the American Academy of Orthopedic Surgeons (AAOS), the European Paediatric Orthopaedic Society (EPOS), and many other medical organizations worldwide. And techniques in the Ponseti method that were developed to treat clubfoot are now being used for other foot problems. For example, stretching and casts show promise in treating congenital vertical talus (CVT). With this condition, which occurs at birth, the foot is also out of alignment but in the opposite way that a clubfoot is out of alignment.

The Ponseti method consists of two main parts: correcting the foot and keeping the clubfoot from coming back (relapsing). Correcting the foot usually takes six to ten weeks. During this time, most babies need to wear five to seven casts and visit the doctor about once a week, though severe cases can take longer to correct. At each visit, the doctor gently stretches the foot and then applies a cast to hold the correction. This process is called serial casting. Though the Ponseti method minimizes surgery, most children need an Achilles (heelcord) tenotomy so that the heel can drop down before they wear their final cast. The tenotomy procedure is explained in the section "Lengthening the Achilles Tendon (Percutaneous Achilles Tenotomy)" on page 37. After the foot is corrected, the child wears a brace to keep the clubfoot from relapsing. If a relapse occurs, the foot must be corrected again with stretching and casts before the child can return to wearing the brace.

Even for difficult cases, stretching and casts are used to correct the foot as much as possible before other surgeries are considered. The Ponseti method includes guidelines for when to consider surgery based on the age of the child and the specific problem with the foot. See Chapter 7, "Surgery," on page 98.

Treatment for clubfoot is very similar whether both feet are affected (bilateral) or only one foot is affected (unilateral). The main difference is that with a unilateral clubfoot, only the affected foot is stretched and put into a cast, and when the child wears a brace the normal foot is positioned at a different angle than the clubfoot.

Finding a Clubfoot Specialist

If your child is diagnosed with clubfoot, you will probably be referred to a doctor who is in the same group as your child's pediatrician. Common practice in referrals varies from one location to another. Some hospitals and clinics have clubfoot teams or groups, but that is not always the case. Before your child starts treatment, it is important to locate a doctor who is trained in and skilled at treating clubfoot with the Ponseti method. Skill at treating clubfoot with this method, which minimizes surgery, is more important than whether the doctor is a pediatric orthopedic doctor or a podiatrist.

- Ask the doctor how many cases of clubfoot they have treated and what the success rate is. Skilled practitioners of the Ponseti method have a success rate of about 95 percent for correcting clubfoot with no surgery beyond a percutaneous Achilles tenotomy. This procedure is explained later in the book in the section "Lengthening the Achilles Tendon (Percutaneous Achilles Tenotomy)" on page 37.

- For help finding a Ponseti-trained doctor, you can contact the Ponseti Clubfoot Center or visit the nosurgery4clubfoot online group for parent recommendations. These organizations are listed in "Clubfoot Information and Support Groups" on page 135 in the Resources chapter.

One parent has this to say about the process of seeking out a doctor skilled in treatment with the Ponseti method:

A lot of doctors say they practice the Ponseti technique but…it's difficult to get them to describe specific training in the Ponseti technique that they or their cast techs have, and how much experience they have treating clubfoot with the technique. Ask specifically about experience with the Ponseti technique and not with just treating clubfoot in general. **[SUZAN]**

Getting a Second Opinion
from the Ponseti Clubfoot Center

The Ponseti Clubfoot Center is located at the University of Iowa Children's Hospital. For a second opinion, you can mail or email photos of your child's feet, or you can travel to Iowa to have your child seen. A doctor at the Ponseti Clubfoot Center will see a child with clubfoot regardless of the family's ability to pay, and they will recommend treatment.

Note: The Ponseti International Association (PIA), which is also located at the University of Iowa, is a nonprofit organization dedicated to best practices in clubfoot treatment for all babies and children. PIA provides funding for the Ponseti Clubfoot Center" and many other clubfoot treatment projects worldwide.

Tamesin offers this advice to parents who are seeking a second opinion for their child's clubfoot treatment:

Before [getting] a second opinion I wrote down everything that had happened to Jasper's feet. I answered questions asked and had a list of questions for the doctor such as:

- How often do you see relapses?
- How often do you suggest ATTT?[1]
- How have you found the Ponseti method? Do you do anything differently?
- What challenges do you find for older children?

---

[1] ATTT is a surgery that is sometimes used to balance ligaments in the foot.

I also asked whether the doctor would look at Jasper's feet and comment on the correction [and] on what he would do if he felt something was needed.

[If your child has atypical clubfoot] you may want to ask how many atypical patients the doctor has, if their cases are similar to this one, what the doctor feels is the long-term outcome, what you as a parent could look out for, what complications surgery may have, and if there are activities you can do to minimize [any possible complications]. If you feel bold enough, ask who he respects in the treatment of atypical clubfoot, and if there are any other associated professionals you should follow up with.

I am sure the doctor we saw was quite happy when I finished grilling him and left him to his quieter patients!   [TAMESIN]

In the following quote, one family expresses how happy…and relieved…they were with their decision to change from one doctor to another:

Initially, the doctor who treated Keiran told us that Keiran would not need the tenotomy. I was thrilled, but I have to wonder what he considered "good" dorsiflexion.[2]

We went to [the Ponseti Clubfoot Center in] Iowa, where my suspicions were confirmed. Keiran's feet were not corrected, and he would need the tenotomy. The difference between semicorrected feet without a tenotomy and fully corrected with a tenotomy is just crazy!

Keiran wouldn't have been walking well at all without that tiny pin prick to lengthen his tendon!   [JOCELYN]

Your Child's Treatment Plan

The Ponseti method has very specific guidelines that doctors must follow for the treatment to be effective. The following table can help you determine whether a doctor is following the Ponseti method.

[2] Dorsiflexion refers to the foot's ability to flex upward.

TABLE 2.1. How to Recognize the Ponseti Method

PONSETI METHOD	RED FLAG
Casts are made of plaster and might be reinforced with fiberglass for older children. Each cast covers the entire leg from the toes up to the groin area.	During serial casting, short casts below the knee should not be used. They do not completely stabilize the tibia and talus bones.
Most babies need five to seven casts, with each cast worn for five to seven days. For more difficult cases, more casts might be needed.	• A young baby should not wear the cast longer than a week. • If the doctor has trouble casting an atypical clubfoot, and the foot keeps slipping inside the cast, you might need to find a doctor with more experience successfully treating atypical clubfoot.
• The cast is removed in the morning that the new cast will be applied • When the final cast comes off, the child wears a foot abduction brace (FAB).	• The cast is removed the day before the new cast is applied. • After the final cast comes off, there is a delay before the child is put into a foot abduction brace. These situations can cause the child's foot to lose its correction.
• After each cast, the child's foot looks better. • After the final cast, the foot turns out so the child's foot will have a normal range of motion.	The foot does not improve or looks worse. Get a second opinion.
Most children (about 80 percent) need a percutaneous Achilles tenotomy before the final cast.	The tenotomy is recommended too early instead of waiting until just before the final cast.
The child wears a foot abduction brace (FAB) with a connecting bar until age four or five to keep the clubfoot from coming back.	• Wearing only an ankle–foot orthosis (AFO) does not hold the foot in the right position. • Stopping brace wear before age four or five can lead to a relapse.

Medical Records

You can ask for a copy of your child's medical records. Legally the doctor's office must provide them to you. Though X rays are not usually needed for clubfoot, they can be useful if your child has another condition in addition to the clubfoot that could affect treatment. Also, if you are moving, it is a good idea to get the medical records so that you can provide them to the doctor you select in your new location. It should be noted that for some parents, looking at medical records helps them clarify their child's condition.

Coping with Treatment

Though you might be concerned about treatment, bear in mind that children are resilient. Most likely, your baby will adjust to it sooner than you do. Feeling sad is common. You might be especially sad the first time you see your child in a cast or brace. Even small things, such as baby clothes that won't fit over the cast or brace, can trigger these feelings. Erwan describes how he felt during his daughter Fleur's treatment for clubfoot:

> The whole experience has been like a bungee jump to me: the extreme fear prior to the jump, the quick-fire ups and downs that follow, and the feeling everything will be all right. I am now in the "lowering-the-rope" phase, where all is nice and safe, but the niggly feeling that you haven't landed yet is in there, tickling you, keeping you in the straight and narrow, no deviation, no sudden moves. Just do what you have to do!   **[ERWAN]**

As your baby or child goes through treatment, take the time to enjoy and admire them. Remember that there is more to your little one than clubfoot. Do some activities that are based on what your child can do, rather than focusing on any temporary limitations during treatment. Nicki has this to say to parents:

For all of you just starting the [clubfoot] journey, take heart. You are doing the best thing possible for your child. You're not taking the easy way out. Swell with pride. Hug that kid. And know that it's all going to be okay. It's not really all that hard. Don't worry. **[NICKI]**

Communicating with Doctors

It is important to understand what your child's treatment will be, how it will help your child, and what you must do for the treatment to be effective. Your doctor should always be willing and able to explain your child's treatment to you.

Medical treatment for a baby or young child can be stressful for families. Parents sometimes disagree or argue about the cause of the clubfoot and the need for treatment. It might help if both parents are able to talk to the doctor and ask questions about any areas of confusion. If only one parent can visit the doctor's office, try to schedule it at a time when the other parent can phone in and join the conversation on a speakerphone or cell phone.

Ask your doctor the following questions in regard to your child's situation. The answers you receive will help you understand your child's treatment:

- Why is this treatment needed?
- How long does the treatment usually last?
- What is the best possible outcome of this treatment? And what is the worst possible outcome?
- Is my child in pain? Do they need pain relief now?

In most cases of clubfoot, a baby is not in pain. However if a child is standing or walking with untreated clubfoot, it can be painful. If this is the case, discuss pain relief for your child. For children who need surgery, anesthesia and pain relief medicines are used.

If you do not understand your child's doctor or are uncomfortable with the care that your child is receiving, bring up the questions or talk about the problems that concern you. Some people find this very difficult to do, but it is worth making the effort. Learn more about diagnosis and treatment or get a second opinion so that you feel comfortable with your child's treatment.

How Doctors Talk about Clubfoot

Each case of clubfoot is unique. That said, there are some medical terms that doctors use to describe aspects of this condition. Learning these terms will help you understand your child's clubfoot and the treatment that is needed. This section explains terms that you are likely to come across. They are listed in alphabetical order. The Glossary contains many more medical terms. See "Glossary" on page 126.

Abduction and Adduction

The terms *abduction* and *adduction* are opposites. Abduction means moving a limb outward away from the center, or midline, of the body. Adduction means moving a limb inward toward the center, or midline, of the body. When correcting the clubfoot, the goal is to gradually stretch the foot into an abducted position (outward) to allow a normal range of motion.

Cavus

A *cavus* is a very high arch. Although some people have normal feet with naturally high arches, the cavus or high arch present in clubfoot is due to a misaligned bone in the foot.

Equinus, Dorsiflexion, and Plantarflexion

The three terms *equinus*, *dorsiflexion*, and *plantarflexion* are often discussed together because they are interrelated. An untreated clubfoot has equinus, which is the heel's tendency to stay up high. This limits or prevents the child from flexing the foot upward. Dorsiflexion refers to how far the foot can flex upward. Plantarflexion is how far the foot can move downward in a pointed-toe position. Dorsiflexion and plantarflexion are measured in degrees from a neutral, flat position called plantigrade (see Figure 2.1).

Doctors treating a baby for clubfoot aim for 10 to 15 degrees of dorsiflexion (upward movement) in a corrected foot. More flexibility is even better, but it might not be achievable in every foot. Less than

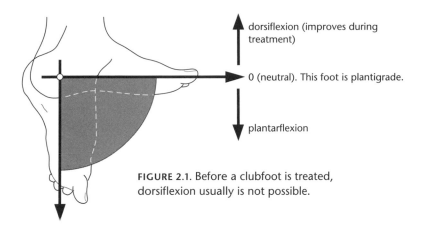

dorsiflexion (improves during treatment)

0 (neutral). This foot is plantigrade.

plantarflexion

FIGURE 2.1. Before a clubfoot is treated, dorsiflexion usually is not possible.

10 degrees of dorsiflexion affects the way the child walks. If your child has only one clubfoot, the other foot could have up to 30 degrees or more of dorsiflexion.

Hypotonia (Low Muscle Tone)

Hypotonia, or low muscle tone, means that a muscle is weaker than normal. Some low muscle tone can occur with clubfoot. For example, the calf muscle of the clubfoot has fewer muscle fibers than usual, resulting in a thinner, higher calf. Temporary low muscle tone can also occur during casting and during bracing when the foot is immobilized. For this reason, the number of hours that older babies and toddlers wear the brace is reduced to twelve to fourteen hours per day. Most of the time spent in the brace is while the child sleeps. This allows time for the child to crawl, walk, and move as usual without the brace, which allows them to build muscle strength.

Manipulation

In the context of clubfoot treatment, *manipulation* means stretching the foot and moving it into a more normal alignment.

Metatarsus Adductus

With metatarsus adductus (MA), the foot is curved so that it bends inward from the middle of the foot to the toes. This condition can range from mild to severe. Severe MA can resemble clubfoot, but doctors can tell these conditions apart because a clubfoot is out of alignment in more ways than a foot with MA. (See "Physical Exam for Clubfoot" on page 6.) If the child's foot is flexible, MA often corrects itself when a child learns to walk.

Ossification

Ossification is the natural process of bones hardening as a baby or child grows older. In young babies, many bones in their bodies are soft. Before these bones ossify, they are more like cartilage than solid bone.

Plantigrade

Plantigrade means that the sole of the foot is flat on the floor when the child is standing.

Positional Clubfoot

With positional clubfoot, the foot has the appearance of a clubfoot but is flexible and easily moves to normal alignment. This condition is caused by the position of the baby's foot before birth. Many doctors do not consider this to be true clubfoot.

Remodeling

In a medical context, *remodeling* refers to an ongoing, normal process in which new bone gradually grows and old bone tissue is absorbed. This is how doctors and nurses sometimes describe the process of improving the shape of bones during clubfoot treatment. For example, the doctor might mention remodeling when talking about the tarsal bones of the foot. When these bones are aligned normally, they tend to grow into the correct shapes. If clubfoot is not treated, the tarsal bones grow into the wrong shapes (they become more deformed).

Supination

Supination is movement in the middle of the foot where the subtalar joint is located. To feel the movement that occurs with clubfoot, stand barefoot on the floor and shift your weight to the outside of your feet. Your big toes might come up off the floor when you do this. The direction this joint tends to move depends on individual foot structure.

Varus and Valgus

The words *varus* and *valgus* are opposites. *Varus* means turned inward toward the midline of the body. *Valgus* means turned outward away from the midline of the body. Figure 2.2 illustrates these two concepts.

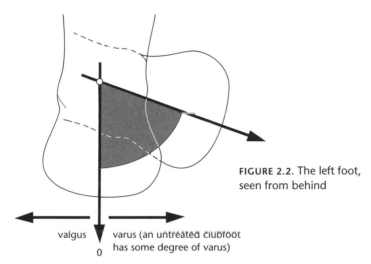

FIGURE 2.2. The left foot, seen from behind

valgus   varus (an untreated clubfoot
   0   has some degree of varus)

If Clubfoot Is Only Part of the Picture

Though clubfoot is usually idiopathic, meaning that its cause is unknown and there may be nothing else wrong with the child, other medical conditions can occur together with clubfoot. This section describes some of these conditions and how doctors typically approach treatment of multiple conditions. These syndromes account for a small minority of all clubfoot cases. They are listed here in alphabetical order.

Amniotic Band Syndrome

Amniotic band syndrome, also called amniotic band constriction syndrome or ABS, is a rare congenital problem that occurs before a baby is born. The baby becomes entangled with strands of the mother's amniotic sac. This most often affects fingers, toes, or limbs. If the feet are constricted, this can be associated with clubfoot.

Arthrogryposis

Arthrogryposis, also called arthrogryposis multiplex congenita (AMC), includes a group of disorders in which there are multiple joint contractures throughout the body that are present at birth. A muscle contracture means that a muscle is tight like a clenched fist and cannot easily relax. This causes the joints to stay in a bent position with a limited range of motion. There are specific types of arthrogryposis such as distal arthrogryposis.

The Ponseti method can be used to treat clubfoot for a baby who has AMC, even if the clubfoot is very severe or the baby has atypical clubfoot. This treatment does not need to be delayed. The Ponseti method should be used to correct the foot as much as possible before any surgeries are considered. From nine to fifteen casts could be needed to correct the foot. Children with AMC have more of a tendency to relapse. One theory as to why this occurs is that they are born with muscle fibers that are tight around a joint.

Look for an experienced doctor who is comfortable treating a child with AMC. If your local doctor is unfamiliar with this process, they might be able to recommend someone with this type of specialized knowledge. Also check with the Ponseti Institute at the University of Iowa or with the nosurgery4clubfoot online group for suggestions from other parents. (See "Clubfoot Information and Support Groups" on page 135.)

Connective-Tissue Disorders

Most people with clubfoot do not have connective-tissue disorders. However, some people with connective-tissue disorders such as Larsen syndrome or Marfan syndrome are prone to clubfoot, hip dysplasia, and dislocated joints. This is due to problems with the soft tissue that connects the joints. Because these syndromes can result in malformed joints, a geneticist might order a skeletal survey. This is a series of X rays to examine the child's bone and joint structure. Treatment for clubfoot with a connective-tissue disorder is mostly the same as treatment for clubfoot alone. If the child is very flexible, the doctor might change the angle of the foot during bracing or modify the brace-wear schedule.

Fibular Hemimelia

Fibular hemimelia is a condition in which the bone in the leg called the fibula is shorter than usual or missing. It can be associated with short stature or a leg-length discrepancy (which means one leg is shorter than the other). This condition might not be noticed until a child is two or three years of age. Treatment for clubfoot in a child with fibular hemimelia is typically the same as treatment for clubfoot alone.

Hip Dysplasia

Hip dysplasia is a condition in which the ball at the top of the thigh bone is not in the correct position inside the hip socket or can easily move into the wrong position. All babies are routinely checked for hip dysplasia. A child with hip dysplasia needs treatment to correct the problem, which can range from mild to severe. Most young babies with hip dysplasia are treated with the Pavlik harness. Some older babies wear a brace called a hip abduction orthosis. Other children need surgery to correct hip dysplasia. If a child has both hip dysplasia and clubfoot, these conditions can often be treated simultaneously. For example, the doctor might begin by having the baby wear a Pavlik harness, and then, when they have adjusted to the harness, start serial casting for clubfoot. For babies or children in a spica cast, the doctor can remove the cast below the knee, stretch the feet, and begin serial casting.

Nerve or Spine Problems

Nerve problems and problems with the spinal cord can affect clubfoot treatment. A child with clubfoot and nerve damage could have feet that tend to relapse more than usual. As these children grow older, some undergo surgery. (See "Posterior Tibial Tendon Transfer (PTTT) for Neuromuscular Clubfoot" on page 106.) Spina bifida, also called myelomeningocele, is a birth defect in which the spinal cord is open. This can be corrected with surgery. In some cases there is also nerve damage, which cannot be repaired. A tethered spinal cord can also be called "closed" spina bifida. Some babies have a neurogenic problem that includes a tethered spinal cord, clubfoot, and hip dysplasia. The neurosurgery department and pediatric orthopedic department work together to develop a course of treatment. A pediatric neurosurgeon must correct the problem with the spinal cord first. Usually, the clubfoot is treated next, followed by the hip dysplasia.

Rocker-bottom Flat Foot

Rocker-bottom flat foot can be a complication arising from failed attempts to correct a clubfoot, especially if the foot is atypical. Rocker-bottom flat foot can be corrected with the Ponseti method. Treatment is difficult, so seek out a skilled doctor with experience in this area.

Note: Rocker-bottom flat foot, also called congenital vertical talus (CVT), can also occur at birth, but not in a baby with clubfoot. With rocker-bottom flat foot, the foot is out of alignment in the opposite way that a clubfoot is out of alignment.

Health-care Workers: Who Does What?

During treatment for your child, you will come in contact with health-care professionals. This section explains the training and role of many of the health-care workers who might be involved in your child's care. Treatment plans vary, so you might not meet all of the types of health-care workers listed here.

Anesthesiologist or Pediatric Anesthesiologist

An anesthesiologist is a doctor who has completed an internship and residency in anesthesiology and is certified by the American Board of Anesthesiologists. A pediatric anesthesiologist has additional training in using anesthesia for babies and children.

Geneticist

A geneticist is a doctor who has studied genetics and is certified by the American Board of Medical Genetics. A pediatric geneticist also completes a residency in pediatrics and is certified by the American Board of Pediatrics. If your child's clubfoot could be associated with a genetic condition or syndrome, you might see a geneticist.

Nurse Practitioner

A registered nurse with at least a master's degree, specialized training, and certifications to perform health examinations and prescribe medications is known as a nurse practitioner (NP). Pediatric NPs specialize in the care of children.

Orthotist

An orthotist makes and fits orthopedic braces prescribed by doctors. Some orthotists are part of a pediatric orthopedic practice. In other cases, the orthotist has an independent practice or works in an orthotic and prosthetic facility.

Pediatric Orthopedic Surgeon

A pediatric orthopedic surgeon specializes in bone and joint problems in babies and children. This doctor completed an orthopedic surgery residency and also completed additional training in pediatric orthopedics.

Pediatrician

A pediatrician is a doctor who specializes in treating children. Most pediatricians are members of professional organizations such as the American Academy of Pediatrics

Pediatric Physical Therapist

A physical therapist (PT) is trained to prevent the onset, or reduce the progression, of conditions resulting from disease, injury, or other causes. A pediatric PT specializes in children.

Physician's Assistant

A physician's assistant (PA) is a licensed health-care professional who provides health-care services under the supervision of doctors. In some states, PAs may prescribe some medications.

Podiatrist

A podiatrist (doctor of podiatric medicine, or DPM) specializes in diagnosing, treating, and preventing foot problems.

Radiologist

A radiologist is trained to interpret X rays. Some diagnostic radiologists are also trained in ultrasound and magnetic resonance imaging (MRI).

Health Insurance and Financial Assistance

Whether or not your child has health insurance, spend some time finding out what expenses will be involved in your child's treatment. Some tips for dealing with health insurance and support organizations are provided in this section. Contact information for these organizations is located in the "Resources" chapter. (See "Financial Assistance" on page 137.)

Some medical expenses might be tax deductible. Tax laws vary from year to year and depend on your individual circumstances. If you must travel a lot for your child's treatment, check with your tax preparer or the appropriate government tax agencies to see if the travel costs, meals, and mileage associated with that travel are tax deductible.

Air and Ground Transportation

Air Care Alliance, Angel Flight, and the National Patient Travel Center provide free or reduced-cost transportation for patients in the United States. For example, one mother flew with Angel Flight from Ohio to Iowa and back every five days for her baby's serial casting at no charge. She was able to make the trip and return in the same day.

Early Intervention Services

The Federal Individuals with Disabilities Education Act (IDEA) requires states to provide early intervention services to eligible children and families. Children with clubfoot who need physical therapy typically qualify for these services. Each state has a separate organization, so you need to contact the one for your location. Most states have programs geared for children who enter treatment from birth to age three, but many children continue with treatment after age three.

Health Insurance

When working with insurance companies, understand your policy, stay organized, and keep records. Keep copies of authorization numbers and referrals. If your child's case is mild and treatment is straightforward, this could be a simple process. For more complicated cases, you might find that paperwork gets lost, something is not filed correctly, the wrong amount is paid, or nothing is paid for a procedure or item that is covered by your policy. As aggravating as this is, stay calm if you can, and contact the insurance company in a timely manner to correct the problem. If you need to call the insurance company, ask for a supervisor or manager. Write down their name and phone number in case you need to reach them again in the future.

If you are struggling with an insurance company, try asking for help from the doctor's office, the orthotics facility, or the hospital where your child was treated. The medical staff might be willing to contact the insurance company about the item or procedure in question. Note that many shoes worn with the foot abduction brace are technically called ankle–foot orthoses (AFOs) and might be considered durable goods, not shoes. If the insurance company still refuses to cover an item necessary to your child's treatment, such as a brace, then you can appeal. Ask for a case manager and find out what the appeals process is.

Military Families with TriCare

TriCare is a health-care program of the United States Department of Defense Military Health System. This section is based on advice provided by parents from military families.

Contact the doctor's office to see if they accept TriCare, and if they are a network provider or a contracted TriCare provider. You can check the TriCare website for your region for a list of network providers. One of the parents in the nosurgery4clubfoot group recommended sending the following items to TriCare when filing a claim for a clubfoot brace:

- A completed TriCare claim form.
- An invoice from MD Orthopaedics if you ordered directly from them. In some cases you should go through Hanger instead of directly to MD Orthopaedics. Check with TriCare first.
- A copy of the doctor's prescription for the brace.
- A copy of the doctor's letter of necessity. Ideally, there should be a sentence in the letter noting that the AFOs (ankle–foot orthoses, which are shoes that go with the brace) and the bar must be replaced as needed due to the child's growth. If you have it, you

can use the same letter each time your child outgrows the brace or shoes.

It is a good idea to make copies of these documents before mailing in the paperwork in case you need to refer to them later.

Ponseti International Association

Due to the support of the Ponseti International Association (PIA), patients with clubfoot can be seen at the Ponseti Clubfoot Center at University of Iowa, Department of Orthopaedic Surgery, regardless of their family's financial situation. The PIA teaches doctors worldwide. The organization's goal is to train doctors in every country so that all children in the world can be treated (about 200,000 children are affected each year).[3]

Ronald McDonald House Charities

The Ronald McDonald House Charities provide a number of services for children. The most well known of these are the Ronald McDonald Houses. These houses are located near children's hospitals in cities and towns in many countries. Families with children in treatment can stay at a Ronald McDonald house at little or no cost. In many cases help is available with meals and transportation to and from the hospital while you are staying at a Ronald McDonald House. Each house has guidelines for guests such as for cleaning the room or suite in which they are staying. For more detailed information, contact the Ronald McDonald House located nearest your destination.

Shriners Hospitals for Children

Shriners Hospitals for Children are associated with the Shriners organization. Some locations have a stronger clubfoot treatment program than others. Shriners hospitals do not charge for treatment. If your child has health insurance, they cover the portion of the treatment costs that insurance does not. If your child has poor health insurance or no health insurance, the hospital will still accept the child for treatment. Doctors there will provide a second opinion, even if

---

[3] Ponseti International Association, "About Us," http://www.ponseti.info/v1/index .php?option=com_content&task=view&id=1&Itemid=44 (accessed 25 October 2011).

you do not choose to use that hospital for treatment. If you do not live near a Shriners hospital, the Shriners organization often is able to arrange transportation for you.

Texas Scottish Rite Hospital for Children

Texas Scottish Rite Hospital for Children provides orthopedic treatment for Texas children, regardless of the ability to pay. Clubfoot treatment with either the Ponseti method or in a French physical therapy program is available. This hospital was founded by the Masons and is not associated with Shriners Hospitals for Children.

Family and Medical Leave Act

In the United States, depending on the size of the company for which you work, the Family and Medical Leave Act (FMLA) might allow you to take up to twelve weeks of unpaid leave per year to care for a family member. This is the same act that covers maternity leave. If your child needs surgery and you can afford to take the time off, this can be helpful while the child is recovering.

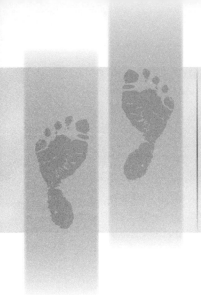

3

Correcting Your Child's Foot

This chapter explains the Ponseti method and describes what doctor visits are like during the first phase of treatment, which is called serial casting.

Figure 3.1 below shows an overview of the Ponseti method.

Note: Treatment is somewhat different for older children. See "Beginning Clubfoot Treatment with an Older Child" on page 44.

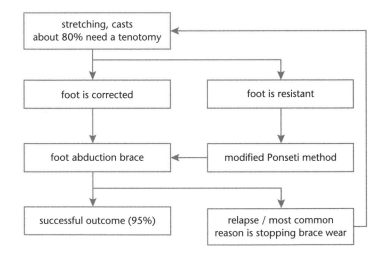

FIGURE 3.1. Overview of the Ponseti method

It is important to find a doctor who is trained in the Ponseti method. The Ponseti International Association provides a list of trained doctors, though some trained doctors are not listed at the website. The nosurgery4clubfoot online group also has a list of doctors recommended by parents. Both of these organizations are listed in "Clubfoot Information and Support Groups" on page 135. Note that this chapter describes what happens at the doctor's office. For suggestions about managing your child at home, see Chapter 4, "Your Child's Casts at Home," on page 51.

Serial Casting

Serial casting is the first phase of treatment in the Ponseti method of treatment for clubfoot. The doctor uses gentle stretching to move the foot into a more normal position. A plaster cast is applied to hold the foot in place (see Figure 3.2). The baby wears the cast for five to seven days. At the next visit the cast is removed, the foot is stretched

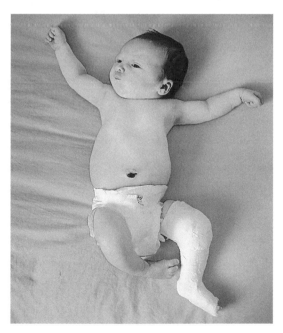

FIGURE 3.2. Farley wearing a cast *(Photo courtesy of Nicki Dugan)*

again, and a new cast is applied. This process is repeated until the foot is fully corrected. Most babies need five to seven casts, but some cases require more.

Figure 3.3 shows a series of casts that are typical of the kind used when a clubfoot is corrected with the Ponseti method. Based on the shape of the casts, you can see how the position of the foot changes during this treatment.

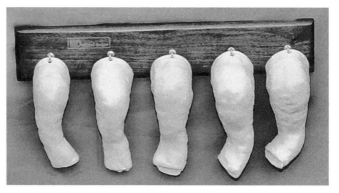

FIGURE 3.3. Model of casts for clubfoot treatment
(Photo courtesy of MD Orthopaedics, Inc.)

About 80 percent of children need an Achilles (heel cord) tenotomy so that the heel can drop before the final cast is applied. If your child has a tenotomy, they will wear the final cast for about three weeks. When the final cast is removed, your child wears a brace to keep the clubfoot from coming back (see Chapter 5, "Wearing a Clubfoot Brace," on page 64).

Why Long-Leg Plaster Casts Are Used

The Ponseti method specifies plaster casts that cover the entire leg from the toes to the groin. Plaster casts are recommended because they are less expensive and because they can be molded more precisely than fiberglass. The knee is bent in the cast to help the foot stay in a flexed position. Each cast must cover the whole leg.

A short cast that comes up only to the knee does not hold the foot in the ideal position. Specifically, a short-leg cast does not stabilize the leg's tibia bone, which affects the position of the talus bone in the foot. This prevents the treatment from working effectively. For older children, the plaster cast can be reinforced with a fiberglass covering to make the cast stronger. This is especially useful for children who are walking.

Your Baby's First Treatment and Cast

Treatment usually starts within two weeks of birth. It is most effective before the baby is nine months of age but can be quite effective up to twenty-eight months of age, and it can be beneficial even for older children.

What to Bring with You to the Appointment

- Supplies for breastfeeding or bottlefeeding.
- A pacifier or comfort object if your child uses one.
- A hand towel with which to wrap the cast on the way home. The towel helps keep plaster flakes from getting all over the car. It also absorbs moisture, which can help the cast dry faster.

Note: When wearing casts, most babies and children fit into the same car seats that they were using before the casts were applied. However, if you find that you need a larger car seat, the Graco Safe Seat is for children up to thirty pounds. Parents have also had good luck with Britax car seats. These models are bigger and longer than some other car seats, so there is more room for the casts and for the foot abduction brace that is worn after the casts.

How the Doctor Stretches the Foot

Stretching the foot does not hurt the baby and works best when the baby is relaxed. The process goes something like this:

1. First, you calm the baby. Breastfeeding or bottlefeeding works well. You might be able to hold your baby while the doctor stretches their foot.

2. The doctor holds the baby's foot and feels for the talus bone, which forms the bottom part of the ankle joint (see Figure 3.4 on the following page).

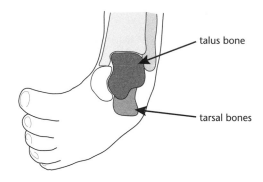

FIGURE 3.4. The tarsal bones next to the talus are out of alignment.

3. The doctor holds the baby's foot steady and massages it to gently stretch the muscles and tendons enough so that it can be moved into a better position (see Figure 3.5).

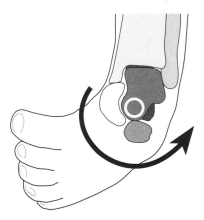

FIGURE 3.5. The white circle shows the talus bone, which does not move. The other tarsal bones pivot around the talus into a better alignment as the doctor corrects the foot.

The foot moves outward, which is called abduction. The doctor stretches the foot only as far as it easily moves outward.

Applying the Cast

Parents can stay with the child while the cast is put on. To apply the cast, two people such as a doctor and a nurse work together (see Figure 3.6).

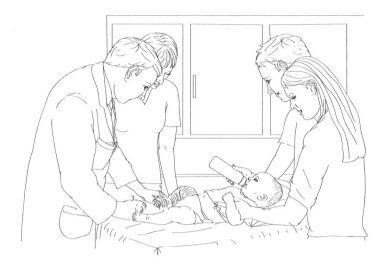

FIGURE 3.6. You can stay with your child when the cast is applied.

The nurse or health-care worker holds the child's foot in its straighter position with the child's knee bent at a 90-degree angle.

The appointment goes something like this:

1. The doctor applies the plaster cast, working from the foot up the leg. The cast covers the whole leg and most of the foot except the tops of the toes.

2. The edges of the cast are trimmed, and padding is added to the top of the cast to protect the skin on the thigh from irritation.

3. You are given instructions about how to care for your child while they are wearing the cast. Generally the instructions are similar to the ones in "Cast Care Instructions" on page 51.

4. You will need to make an appointment to return to see the doctor in five to seven days for the next treatment and cast.

How Your Child's Foot Improves Inside the Cast

As babies and children grow, new bone is created in their bodies. This is a natural process called remodeling. The shapes a child's bones grow into are affected by how the bones are used and by the pressure of surrounding cartilage and adjacent bones and joints.

While your child is in the cast, the tarsal bones, cartilage, and joints continue to grow and remodel into more normal shapes because they are in better alignment. This happens faster with young babies but occurs for all children who are still growing. The muscles and ligaments get used to the new position of the foot. When the cast comes off, the foot looks better. The high arch of the foot, also called the cavus, is the area where you can see the changes first.

Hammertoes or "Curly Toes"

Tight ligaments in the toes can cause hammertoes—sometimes called curly toes. These toes bend upward in the middle instead of lying flat. Hammertoes are common in kids with clubfeet but can also occur in normal feet. As some babies and children undergo treatment for clubfoot, their toes move into unusual positions. They usually resolve on their own with time. If a child does not outgrow hammertoes, the toes can be stretched, or if necessary, the tendons to the toes can be released with surgery so that the toes lie flat.

Ongoing Treatments and Cast Changes

Your child wears each cast until the day that the next cast will be applied. If the cast is removed too soon, such as the day before your doctor visit, the correction that was achieved by the cast can be lost. In other words, the clubfoot will begin to come back. This is called a relapse. Because the muscles and tendons on the inside of the foot and calf are stronger than the ones on the opposite side, they tend to pull the foot back into the clubfoot position.

The original Ponseti method specified soaking the cast in water to soften it and then removing it with a cast cutter. Though the Ponseti Clubfoot Center still uses this method, in many facilities, a healthcare worker or doctor removes the cast with a cast saw (see Figure 3.7) because it is quicker. The cast saw is designed for safe use, and a skilled practitioner can use one to remove the plaster cast without hurting even a young baby.

After the cast comes off, your child's skin is checked for any irritated areas and is washed. The baby is calmed, and the doctor stretches the foot outward for about a minute. Then the next cast is

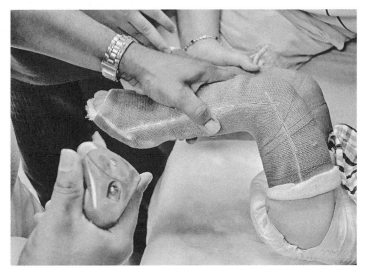

FIGURE 3.7. A cast saw *(Photo courtesy of Matthew Dobbs, MD)*

applied. This process is repeated until the foot can easily stretch outward to the side about 60 degrees. About 80 percent of children need an Achilles tenotomy so that the heel can drop downward before the final cast is applied. This is described in "Lengthening the Achilles Tendon (Percutaneous Achilles Tenotomy)" below.

Immunizations

Wearing casts does not have to interfere with a child's scheduled immunizations. Regular shots such as two-month immunizations can usually be given above the casts. If your child has a history of reacting to shots and you want to postpone them until after the casts are removed, discuss this with your child's doctor.

Lengthening the Achilles Tendon (Percutaneous Achilles Tenotomy)

The Achilles tendon is located in the back of the heel (see Figure 3.8 on the following page). This tendon is not as flexible as the ligaments and muscles that the doctor stretches during serial casting. When the Achilles tendon is very short and tight, the heel cannot move down far enough for the child to put their foot flat when standing. For this reason, most babies with clubfoot need surgery to release this ten-don. This surgery is called a percutaneous tenotomy (cutting of a tendon through the skin) of the Achilles tendon. Based on medical research in older children who were treated for clubfoot, no weak-ness in the foot is associated with a percutaneous Achilles tenotomy.

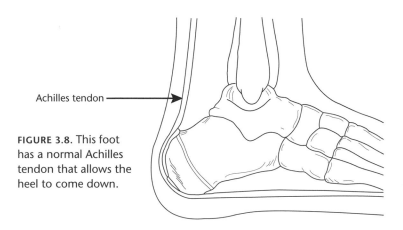

Achilles tendon ⎯⎯⎯⎯⎯⎯

FIGURE 3.8. This foot has a normal Achilles tendon that allows the heel to come down.

The tenotomy is very quick and has been described by some par-ents as a "poke" to the back of the heel. The Achilles tendon will re-attach over a period of two to three weeks while the baby is in the cast. The traditional Ponseti method specifies local anesthesia for babies for pain relief during the tenotomy. A shot with pain relief medicine is given in the baby's heel. The baby is awake and does not have to re-cover from the effects of general anesthesia. Usually the tenotomy is done in the doctor's office.

Older children who begin treatment later or who are experienc-ing a relapse might have light general anesthesia instead. If your child will be put to sleep for the surgery, you will be given instructions from your doctor's office or hospital about how to prepare your child for surgery. For more topics regarding general anesthesia and sur-gery in a hospital, see Chapter 7, "Surgery," on page 98.

How the Doctor Does the Tenotomy

During this visit, the doctor measures the child's feet so the brace can be prescribed and ordered. The brace is called a foot abduction orthosis (FAB). Measuring for and ordering the brace now allows enough time to receive it before the final cast comes off.

The tenotomy procedure typically goes like this:

1. For an office visit with local anesthesia, the baby is calmed. Breastfeeding or bottle-feeding is recommended for this purpose.

2. The baby or child is given pain relief by one of these methods:
   - For an office visit with local anesthesia, the baby is given a shot in the heel. This shot numbs the area and is similar to the medicine that a dentist uses.
   - If the baby or child will be put to sleep, anesthesia is given as described in the section "Anesthesia" on page 101.

3. The doctor uses a very thin scalpel to cut the Achilles tendon (see Figure 3.9). This small cut usually does not leave a scar. Stitches are not needed.

4. The baby's foot and leg are put into a cast. There is a small amount of bleeding from the tenotomy, which might stain the back of the cast. Because the cast is absorbent, the stain could be the size of a quarter or larger. If your child has had general anesthesia, they are moved to the recovery room.

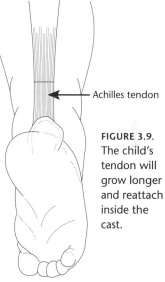

Achilles tendon

FIGURE 3.9. The child's tendon will grow longer and reattach inside the cast.

5. Your doctor advises you about pain relief for your baby during the first day or two after the tenotomy. Often infant drops of acetaminophen (Infant Tylenol) are suggested. Check with your doctor about the recommended dosage for your child.

6. You are given instructions for managing your child in a cast, which is similar to the previous casts. The cast is worn for three weeks.

When Keiran Had His Tenotomies

Jocelyn's son Keiran had tenotomies when he was five weeks old. Though she was scared before the tenotomies, Jocelyn found the experience was much better than she expected. She offers parents some perspective and describes Keiran's tenotomies:

You need to have all your fears about the tenotomy erased! Look at your foot. Flex it upward and run your hand up and down the back of your ankle. What you feel is the Achilles tendon. It is right under the skin and almost feels like bone.

On a clubfoot, the Achilles tendon is too short, as are the muscles around it. When a clubfoot flexes upward, it doesn't go far enough to allow for proper walking. The only way to fix that is to make the tendon longer.

The way they do it is so fast and easy. I was scared, too. Keiran was five months old. They laid him on his back on the table. I was by his head playing with him and talking to him. Maria (Dr. Morcuende's nurse) and another nurse each held a leg.

About five minutes before they started, they applied a numbing agent to the back of the first heel. Then, Dr. Morcuende asked my husband to rub the cleaning solution on Keiran's heel while Maria held Keiran's foot flexed up as far as it would go. She kept pushing up on his heel as Dr. Morcuende poked the Achilles tendon through the skin with a blade the size of a cataract blade (that is teeny tiny... they use it to operate on EYES. It's like a pin prick!).

The tendon made a low pop noise at which point Maria lessened pressure on the heel and applied gauze. It did not bleed very much at all. They casted the foot immediately afterward, flexing the foot up to stretch the calf muscles so that the tendon would grow back at the correct length.

The second foot was exactly the same. Keiran cried some for the first foot, but he fell asleep during the casting and slept through the second foot. It was WAY less scary than I thought it would be.

Those casts stay on three weeks to allow the tendon to fully heal. I can't find any scars from the tenotomies at all, anywhere on either heel. He is ten months old now and doing so great!

[JOCELYN]

Your Child's Corrected Foot

When the final cast comes off, your child's foot turns out, so it might seem overcorrected to you. This is done on purpose so that the child will have a normal range of motion and be comfortable when wearing a brace. If you look at a normal foot, it can move outward to about the position of the final cast.

The doctor examines the foot and applies a foot abduction brace to maintain the correction. The child's foot must be able to comfortably point outward at a 60-degree angle, and the heel must be able to move downward so that it does not slip out of the brace. Now the child is ready to start the next phase of treatment by wearing a brace. (See Chapter 5, "Wearing a Clubfoot Brace," on page 64.)

Relapses

When a clubfoot has been corrected but the problem later returns, the foot has relapsed. The most common reason for relapse is not wearing the brace consistently. If the brace is worn and the foot relapses anyway, it could be due to a growth spurt or muscle imbalances in the foot and stiff ligaments. Relapsed clubfeet can be treated by the Ponseti method of serial casting with an Achilles tenotomy if needed. In this situation, most children need three or four treatments and casts.

In some cases, stretches or physical therapy can help keep a child's foot flexible if it has been corrected but is stiffening up during brace wear. As more research has been done into the rate of relapse, the brace-wear schedule has extended from age two to age four or five. Many doctors see physical therapy as a way to improve flexibility and strength in a child's foot. This can be especially helpful in keeping the tendons stretched if an older child begins to relapse, which can occur during a sudden growth spurt if the Achilles tendon does not keep up with growth in the rest of the foot. In this situation, physical therapy can improve flexibility for some children and make it less likely that they will need a tenotomy or an anterior tibialis tendon transfer (ATTT), surgically moving tendons in the foot. See "Balancing the Ligaments in the Foot with ATTT" on page 102.

How to Tell If a Child's Foot Is Relapsing

When toddlers are learning to stand, they sometimes bear weight on the outside of their feet. This might not be due to a relapse. If your child's foot is still flexible and can move into a normal position, then, given some time and practice, your child will most likely figure out how to better balance himself.

If your child's foot has been corrected, but it begins to move into a clubfoot position, have your child's clubfoot doctor check the foot.

Some signs that a foot is relapsing include:

- The foot is taking on a "C" shape as the forefoot turns inward.
- The foot is less flexible. The heel does not come down as far as it used to.
- The child has an uneven gait and might gallop instead of walking or running.
- The child cannot stand flat footed and, instead, walks on the outside of the foot or on tiptoes.

Note: You can read more about relapsing on the nosurgery4club foot online group site. Go to the hot topics folder and look for relapsing.

Children who have nerve problems or weak muscles in their legs can be more inclined to relapse. In this situation, a child might benefit from physical therapy that targets the weak muscle. Some children who have nerve problems and continuously relapse need ATTT surgery when they are older.

A study at the University of Iowa found that for a small group of children, clubfoot recurs after age five. In these cases, serial casting followed by anterior tibialis tendon transfer (ATTT) surgery gives good results. Though the feet might not look perfect, most people in the study reported that their feet did not limit their activities.

Correcting a Relapsed Clubfoot

The process of stretching and applying casts is basically the same if a foot has relapsed. If your child is old enough to stand or walk, the plaster casts are reinforced with a fiberglass covering to make them more durable.

Many older children crawl or walk while wearing casts, but their muscles do lose some strength. This is normal, and it is temporary. However, because of this, a child who was walking before the casts were put on might not be able to walk afterward until they have had time to regain muscle strength. A rule of thumb is that for every week the child is in the cast, they will need a week of strengthening after the final cast is removed to regain the level of activity that they had before the casts were applied. For example, if the child wears casts for five weeks, then after the final casts are removed, it will take five weeks for them to regain the strength that was lost.

What to Bring with You to the Appointment

- For babies, supplies for breastfeeding or bottlefeeding.
- A pacifier or comfort object if your child uses one.
- For older children, a wagon or stroller. The casts are heavy, so this will make it easier to get your child to the car.
- If your child is old enough to use the bathroom, make a potty stop on your way in to see the doctor.
- A hand towel to wrap the leg cast on the way home. The towel helps keep plaster flakes from getting all over the car. It also absorbs moisture, which can help the cast dry faster.

When Jasper's Feet Relapsed

Tamesin's son Jasper relapsed, and he underwent serial casting at age four for bilateral clubfoot. Here is her account of the experience:

> Recasting was fine as we could explain it to Jasper now that he was a big boy and not that newborn baby who was casted so long ago. The physical therapist (PT) who casted him kept him very involved. She would give him a choice of toys to play with, he would choose which color fiberglass would be used, and he had a special treat on cast days (usually junk—hot chips, fries, or chocolate; his choice). We made it a special day each week. ➡

He did find the manipulations for each new casting quite painful as they really had to stretch his feet since they had stiffened up a lot, but it was not painful about a minute after. Also the PT explained that the electric saw although noisy didn't hurt but tickled instead like a tickling machine. He thought that was great and giggled every time the cast was cut off.

The recovery after the final cast was removed took ages. Jasper ended up in about eight weeks of casting, so his calves, ankles, and forefeet had become weak. It took a while to walk, then a few weeks longer to walk properly without looking all bent over, and longer again before he felt comfortable jumping. The first few weeks after casting were painful. We used mild painkillers para-acetylaminophenol (Panadol) and ibuprofen (Neurofen). Also his feet weren't visually straight after the last cast although they were considered corrected (I traveled 1,000 kilometers to get a second opinion) but about a month of [brace] wear and they straightened up.

Now, almost six months on, his feet look great. As for preschool during casting—he was the star. Everyone wanted casts like Jasper's!

[TAMESIN]

Beginning Clubfoot Treatment with an Older Child

A child who is old enough to walk and has untreated clubfoot will have a large callus on the side of the foot. This is unusual in the United States but is more common in the developing world or in locations where treatment resources are limited. When the child has been walking on clubfeet, some of the bones inside the foot have grown into the wrong shapes. Even in this situation, it is best to begin clubfoot treatment with the Ponseti method. The goal is to correct the foot as much as possible and only then to consider whether surgery is needed.

The Ponseti method is applicable and gets very good results during childhood and adolescence. Children up to the age of 9 or 10 who have relapsed after having foot surgery in infancy or early childhood can still sometimes benefit from the Ponseti method. The Ponseti Clubfoot Center has successfully treated patients up to 18 years old.

The Ponseti treatment method is different for children who begin treatment when they are older. In such cases:

- The average number of casts for children who are over 2 years of age when they begin treatment is about ten.

- The child wears each cast for two weeks (for babies only one week is needed). After the cast dries, the child can stand and walk while wearing the cast.

- The foot will be corrected to 30 to 40 degrees of abduction (turn-out) instead of 70 degrees as is done for babies.

- Physical therapy is especially important in older children to develop and maintain flexibility in their feet.

- Up to age 6, children can wear a foot abduction brace (FAB) to maintain their foot correction. Children older than 6 might need custom ankle–foot orthoses (AFOs). Work with a Ponseti-trained doctor who has experience with these cases.

Adopting a Child with Untreated Clubfoot

Congratulations on the new addition to your family, and kudos to you for taking the clubfoot journey with your child. If you live in a country where clubfoot is treated soon after birth, you might need to do some research to find a doctor who has experience treating clubfoot in older children. Lori Jo's son Noah had already started walking on his untreated clubfoot before he was adopted. She offers this advice about shoes:

While awaiting casting, consider "crib shoes" like Robeez. They are easy to put on and give the child's foot some protection while walking. It is very hard to get a clubfoot into a regular shoe. Noah came to us in high-top shoes, but he had what I'm sure were healed pressure sores on his ankles from shoes that simply didn't fit his foot.

[LORI JO]

Noah's Story

When Lori Jo and her husband adopted Noah, he was twenty-one months old with untreated clubfoot and untreated arthrogryposis (AMC). Here is a photo of Noah's feet before treatment (see Figure 3.10). Noah was walking on the sides of his feet. To keep from falling over, he would continuously rock back and forth when standing.

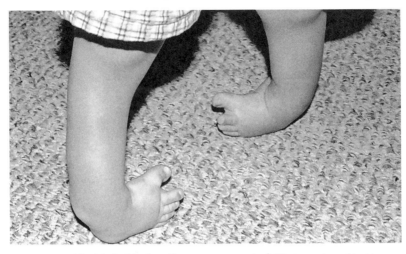

FIGURE 3.10. Noah's feet before they were corrected *(Photo courtesy of Lori Jo Learned-Burton, MD)*

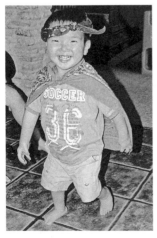

FIGURE 3.11. Noah on the go *(Photo courtesy of Lori Jo Learned-Burton, MD)*

Noah's clubfeet were especially hard to treat because he has AMC, which causes muscle contractures. At his first doctor visit, Noah's feet were so stiff that only his toes moved. Dr. Lund consulted with an expert in Baltimore who had extensive experience treating neglected clubfoot. After eleven casts and a tenotomy, Noah's outcome was extremely successful.

The photo on the left in Figure 3.12 shows Noah's left foot with a callus. The photo on the right shows when the calluses disappeared. Calluses are common in cases of untreated clubfoot.

This callus took two years
to go away!

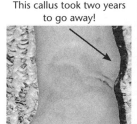
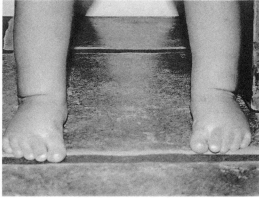

FIGURE 3.12. Noah's left foot is shown with a callus (left). His feet are also shown when the calluses were gone (right). *(Photos courtesy of Lori Jo Learned-Burton, MD)*

In spite of his successful treatment with the Ponseti method, Lori Jo was told by doctors that the Ponseti method would not be effective in treating Noah's feet. One doctor even told her that while Noah was running around in the same room.

Amelia's Story

When she was adopted, Amelia was sixteen months old and had untreated clubfoot. After her feet were corrected with serial casting, one foot relapsed even though she was wearing her brace as directed. To correct the relapse, Amelia underwent additional serial casting (see Figure 3.13 on the next page) followed by ATTT surgery and now wears a brace to maintain the correction.

Amelia was first seen by Dr. V., who stretched her foot and applied a series of four casts. Then she had an Achilles tenotomy and the final cast was applied. Dr. V. moved, and Amelia was seen by a different pediatric orthopedic doctor. Her final casts were removed, and she went into a Denis Browne bar and Markell shoes for twenty-three hours a day. Three months later, her brace wear was reduced to fourteen hours a day. A few months later, her mother, Kim, noticed that Amelia's foot was turning up and that she still had a crease in the bottom of her foot. Kim says:

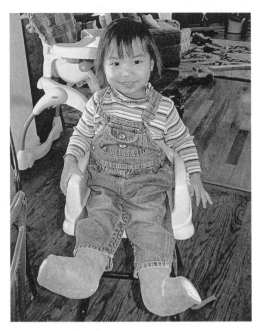

FIGURE 3.13. Amelia wearing casts *(Photo courtesy of Kim Wells)*

I emailed photos to Dr. Ponseti, and he said she was not fully corrected and had no dorsiflexion. After much debate, we decided to go to St. Louis for treatment since it is five hours away and Iowa is over eight hours away. We did not feel comfortable staying in Cincinnati since that doctor was not a Ponseti-certified doctor. He has since been to St. Louis to visit Dr. Dobbs and his staff, which is great for the Cincinnati area.   **[KIM]**

Kim and her husband chose Dr. Dobbs as Amelia's new clubfoot doctor. He ordered an electromyography (EMG), which is a test to identify damaged nerves to see if that might be why Amelia's feet were relapsing. The EMG showed nerve damage in both legs, especially in the left perineal nerve. The test confirmed that Amelia's feet would always have a tendency to lose correction because the nerve damage affects her nerve and muscle control. In this case Dr. Dobbs recommended ATTT surgery (see "Amelia's ATTT Surgery" on page 104), followed by brace wear. Kim has this to say:

> ATTT surgery works well with the children with nerve damage as long as they continue to use the brace as prescribed. There is no reason to not wear that brace. We don't have any issues with Amelia not wanting to wear the brace. **[KIM]**

Older Children During Treatment

When used with older children, the Ponseti method is mainly the same as with younger children, with some adjustments based on the age and size of the child. The Ponseti method specifies long-leg plaster casts during serial casting. For older children, the casts can be reinforced with a fiberglass shell, which protects the cast. Many children crawl or walk in their casts. The casts get dirty but are worn only for a week or two. Lori Jo describes Noah's activities while wearing his casts:

> The casts are bent at the knee, and Noah learned to balance on them by kind of sitting on the back of the upper leg part. He was dancing and running in them in the end. **[LORI JO]**

Plaster casts are heavy. Consider using a stroller, wagon, or wheelchair. It can be difficult to lift and carry an older child. You might be able to get a temporary disabled parking permit from the Department of Motor Vehicles (DMV) while your child is wearing a cast. These placards allow you to park in handicapped parking spaces. (See "Temporary Disabled Parking Placards" on page 59.)

When the Casts Come Off

When children who are old enough to walk wear leg casts, they usually cannot walk at first when they get out of the casts. While they are wearing the cast, they lose muscle tone. When the casts come off, children will be using a different set of muscles to walk normally than they did before. As a general rule, it takes as long as they were in the casts to relearn how to walk. Lori Jo describes her experiences when Noah's casts were removed:

> The local baby pool and a round floatie were lifesavers. It was basically aqua therapy for Noah. The buoyancy helped hold him up and helped him with his balance. Most older kids that were walking on their clubfoot have a huge callus on the side of their foot. It took almost two years for that skin to return to normal once Noah's foot was corrected.   **[LORI JO]**

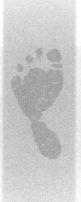
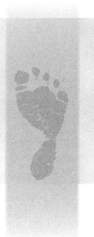

4

Your Child's
Casts at Home

This chapter provides tips and practical suggestions to make it easier to manage at home when your child is wearing a cast. As much as possible, treat your child as you usually do. Your child will sense your attitude. Of course, you should respond if they are in pain or need help, but do not feel as if you have to jump every time they make a sound. Give them a little time to settle, just as you would any other child.

Cast Care Instructions

The doctor provides you with instructions when your child wears a cast. Generally, they are similar to the ones listed here.

- When the cast is new, it should rest on a soft pillow until the plaster dries. A hard surface could dent the cast.

- When your child is on their back, place a pillow under the cast to elevate the leg so the heel is just beyond the pillow. This prevents pressure on the heel.

- Check the circulation in the foot based on the instructions that your doctor or hospital gives you. This is to make sure that the cast is not too tight. Gently squeeze the toe. It should get pale as the blood runs out. When you let go, the toe should regain its color as the blood flows back in. If the toe stays pale for some time, the circulation could be poor.

- Make sure you can see the top of your baby's toes.
- Keep the cast clean and dry. When you diaper your baby, the top of the cast should be outside your baby's diaper.

The doctor applies padding to the top of the cast to protect the baby's skin. You can replace it if it wears away. Mole foam or moleskin adhesive padding is available at most pharmacies or drugstores. You can also apply waterproof tape to the top edge of the cast. Taping the edges makes a smoother surface against your child's skin than the cast. It also adds a barrier in case urine or stool leaks out of the diaper. If the tape gets soiled, it can be removed and replaced with clean tape. Some recommended tapes are listed here:

- Nexcare waterproof tape, available at Walmart and Target stores.
- Hy-Tape, which is pink and sometimes used at hospitals for wound care, or Tegaderm hospital tape.
- If your child is of walking age, you can wrap the bottom of the cast with athletic tape to help keep the cast in one piece.

Causes for Concern

The following situations could indicate a problem with the cast. Call your doctor's office for advice if they occur:

- You have checked the circulation in the foot and are worried that the cast is too tight.
- You cannot see the top of your child's toes, and it seems that the foot has slipped inside the cast.
- You see drainage or smell a foul odor coming from inside the cast.
- The skin is very red or irritated at the edges of the cast.
- Your child has a fever for no apparent reason and does not have a cold or virus.
- Your child seems to be in pain or is inconsolable, and you do not know why.

Though it is normal for a child to fuss while adjusting to the cast, the cast should not be painful.

Caring for Your Baby in a Cast

While your child is in a cast, you will need to make some adjustments to your routine. Your child's plaster cast must be kept dry, which means that baths or showers are not allowed. Here are some suggestions to help with your child's personal hygiene.

Diapering

If possible, ask a nurse to help you practice changing a diaper at the hospital before you take your child home. Change the diaper regularly in order to prevent any wetness from the diaper from wicking into the cast.

Skin Care

Skin irritation is common when children wear a cast. If the skin is irritated, clean it gently with a soft washcloth and apply a diaper cream. If the child's skin becomes very irritated where the edge of the cast rubs, you can tape the cast.

Incisions

An incision is the place where the doctor made a cut such as for a percutaneous Achilles (heel-cord) tenotomy. If your child has an incision, it will not develop a scab. This is normal. The incision is covered by the cast and cannot be seen. The incision usually heals within two weeks. Signs of infection include redness, tenderness, swelling, and fever. If you are concerned about the incision, contact your doctor.

Atypical Clubfoot: Big Toes and Toenails

Many babies with atypical clubfoot have big toes that are larger than usual and stick up in what is called a called hyperextended position. The toenail for the big toe can grow straight upward. As the baby gets older and the clubfoot is corrected, the angle of the big toe and the toenail typically improve. Here are some tips from parents about keeping your child's toenails healthy:

- Gently push down on the toenail at bath time to encourage it to gradually stretch into a more normal alignment.
- Clean the big toenails with hydrogen peroxide.
- Allow your child to go barefoot when they are not wearing the brace.

- Do not cut the toenail too short.
- Allow some room in the toe when putting socks on your child.

If the skin around your child's toenail is irritated or you are worried that it might be infected, contact your child's regular pediatrician.

Older Children in Casts

Toddlers can sit, roll over, crawl, pull to a stand, and cruise while wearing casts. You will probably be able to use the same high chair or booster seat that you have been using. For bathing, you can try a sponge bath on the kitchen counter or on the bathroom floor.

When you lift your child, use care. The cast adds weight, and it can take practice to get used to it.

Here are some suggestions.

- Protect your back by using safe lifting techniques. Bend your knees, and place one arm beneath your child's shoulders and your other arm beneath the buttocks.
- If two people are lifting an older child, one person supports the shoulders while the other lifts the child's legs.
- You can use a stroller or a wagon with pillows to go on walks. Children who are too old for a stroller or wagon might prefer to use a pediatric wheelchair.

When settling your child onto a flat surface, use rolled-up towels or small pillows to support the feet or legs so that the child is comfortable and the edges of the cast do not press against the skin. For example, place rolled-up towels beneath the knees or ankles to support them.

Clothing Tips

Here are some suggestions about clothing from parents:

- Buy clothes a size or two larger than the child would normally wear to fit over the casts.
- Use footed pajamas with some snaps left open.

- At nighttime you can use a sleep sack to keep your child warm (see Figure 4.1). HALO Innovations and BabyHipWear make sleep sacks that work well with casts and braces.

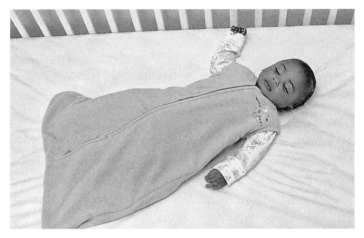

FIGURE 4.1. A SleepSack wearable blanket *(Photo courtesy of HALO Innovations, Inc.)*

- For onesies, you can use Add-a-Size Baby Garment Extenders available through One Step Ahead. These make leg openings bigger.
- Loose dresses help camouflage the casts. Some people will assume that your child is wearing tights, rather than casts.

Tovey offers this advice based on her experience with her son, Jack, who was born with clubfoot:

Jack was my fourth child, and I used everything with him that I did with the other three. I would recommend a high chair with a fully removable tray, and buy nonnewborn clothes with snaps all the way down legs for the bracing phases. During the casting stage, any pants usually fit and even the one-piece footed outfits, but after casting, you can't have feet. Snap legs make it way easier. It is really not bad to find things that work.   **[TOVEY]**

Crawling, Standing, or Walking in a Cast

If your child's cast is made only of plaster, wait until it dries before allowing your child to bear weight. When the cast is damp, pressure from standing or crawling could dent it or affect its shape. If your child's cast is reinforced with fiberglass, then it will quickly dry.

Older babies or children can continue to crawl, stand, or walk while they are wearing casts. Children who walk in casts use different muscle groups from those they will use when the cast is removed. Some of your child's leg muscles will lose muscle tone during treatment with the cast. This is normal, and after the cast is removed, your child will gradually regain muscle tone in those areas.

Comforting a Fussy Child

When your child is in a cast, it is sometimes hard to tell if their fussiness is due to a problem with the cast or some other cause such as teething, a virus, or an ear infection. Here are some things to try:

- Change their diaper. While you are changing your baby, check for any skin irritation or diaper rash.

- If the weather is hot and your child is in a cast, do what you can to cool them off. Dress your child in as little as possible and sponge off their skin with a damp cloth.

- Some children have muscle aches when they stop wearing casts. If you believe your child is in pain, check with your doctor to find the right dosage of pain relief medicine such as acetaminophen (Tylenol) or ibuprofen (Advil) for your child. See the following section, "Pain Management at Home."

Pain Management at Home

During your child's treatment, it is best to discuss pain management for your child with your child's doctor or nurse. Either of these professionals can tell you if pain relief is typically recommended for specific procedures.

If your child is in pain, try to stay calm. This reduces their anxiety and helps you focus on figuring out the source and intensity of the pain. If your child is old enough, ask them where and how much it hurts. For babies or very young children, use behavior and appearance as a guide. A child's age and personality affect how they react to pain. One child might be very quiet, while another screams. Children in pain usually want to stay closer than usual to a parent or primary caregiver. Try to make yourself available. For example, put the baby where they can see you while you make dinner.

Pain also can be treated with nonmedical techniques, such as distraction. Distraction can be as simple as reading them a story, allowing a child to watch more television than usual, playing music that they like, or breastfeeding.

The most common over-the-counter pain relief medications for children are acetaminophen (Tylenol) and ibuprofen (Advil or Motrin). Do not combine these medications unless your doctor has given you instructions to do so.

- Acetaminophen provides pain relief for mild to moderate pain and fever. It does not relieve inflammation. Overdosing a child with acetaminophen can damage the liver and kidneys. Acetaminophen is included in many cough or cold medicines. Read medicine labels carefully to avoid accidentally giving your child too much acetaminophen. Make sure that you have the right-size teaspoon or dropper.

- Ibuprofen is a nonsteroidal anti-inflammatory drug (NSAID). It reduces inflammation, provides pain relief, and reduces fevers. Ibuprofen prevents the body from making prostaglandins (hormones that produce inflammation and pain). As a side effect, ibuprofen can cause stomach irritation. It is best to take ibuprofen on a full stomach. If your child is allergic to aspirin or has asthma, check with your doctor before giving them ibuprofen.

Aspirin is not recommended for babies or children unless directed by a doctor. Aspirin use in children is linked to a rare but serious disease called Reye's syndrome. Naproxen (Aleve, Naprosyn, or Anaprox) is recommended only for children who are at least twelve years old.

Sleeping

The first night after a cast is put on is the hardest, but your baby will adjust to sleeping in it. If your child received general anesthesia during surgery, this could throw off their sleeping schedule for as long as three weeks. Here are some suggestions that might help ease the adjustment period:

- **Use products for pain relief.** Check with the doctor to confirm the best pain medicine and the dose for your child at bedtime. Some doctors recommend infant ibuprofen (Advil or Motrin) or acetaminophen (Tylenol) for pain, or Benadryl to make a child drowsy.

- **Prop up the legs and upper body.** Use a rolled-up blanket or cushion under the child's legs.

- **Try a change of position.** If the baby is old enough, you can put them on their tummy if they are more comfortable sleeping that way. Make sure that the baby can breathe easily and that no blankets are near their face.

- **Consider teething or other problems.** If your child is inconsolable, the problem could be something else (not their feet). Check them for the same things you would normally look for in a fussy baby: teething, symptoms of a virus, or an ear infection.

If you are worried about your child, check with your doctor. Some children don't sleep as well in the cast as they did before.

Your Feelings

At first the idea of caring for a child in a cast can seem like running a slow-motion marathon. Everything takes longer than it ought to, and facing the weeks of treatment ahead is daunting. As you and your child develop routines, life with the cast becomes easier to manage.

Remember that in spite of the fact that your child's feet are the center of your universe now, this will not always be the case. There is far more to your child than their clubfoot and far more to you than being their caretaker, important a job as that is. Take the time to enjoy your child and appreciate your time together.

How Other People React to Your Child

Some people stare when they see a child in a cast or brace. Bear in mind that they are probably trying to figure out what the baby or child is wearing and why. It is up to you whether you want to ignore this or offer a brief explanation. An older child wearing a cast due to a relapse might get embarrassed when people stare. Talk to your child about ways to respond if this happens. In particular, remind them that other children are curious about a child in a cast but are often friendly.

Temporary Disabled Parking Placards

An older child in a cast can be difficult to get in and out of a car. If it is raining and your child is in a plaster cast that is supposed to stay dry, that just adds to the problem. In the United States, while your child is in a cast, you can use a temporary disabled placard. It is good for up to six months and allows you to park in handicapped parking spaces. These spaces have extra room on the sides, so that you won't get pinned in by other cars parking too close for you to get your child out of the car. To get a temporary disabled parking placard, contact the Department of Motor Vehicles (DMV) for your state. You will need to get a form for your child's doctor to sign. When you turn in the signed form at the DMV, you can get the placard. Follow the instructions from the DMV about where to put the placard in your car and when to use it. In some states, this is free. Other states charge a fee for the placard.

Child Care

If your child goes to child care, talk to the provider about your child's treatment. If possible, stay the first time or two that you bring your child into the care center. That will give the child-care provider time to learn how to care for your child and to ask any questions that come up. Here are some suggestions:

- **Casts.** Explain that the casts need to stay dry. Show the child-care provider how to change diapers so that the casts stay clean.

For older children, let the child-care provider know it is all right for your child to crawl or walk while casted.

- **Brace.** Make sure that the provider understands how long the brace must be worn each day. For example, you can bring your child in wearing the brace and ask the child-care provider to remove the brace at noon. If your child is mobile, tell the provider that standing or walking in a brace is okay with the doctor.

Brothers and Sisters

Take the time to talk to all of the children in the family about your child's treatment. Often, older siblings have questions about why treatment is needed. Explain that the treatment can take a long time, but that it is helping the child so that they will not have problems later. Sometimes siblings worry about the child in treatment, especially if that child is fussy. They might feel bad for that child and even cry. Other children might be jealous of the extra attention that a child needs while in treatment. Let your children know that you love everyone in the family just the same.

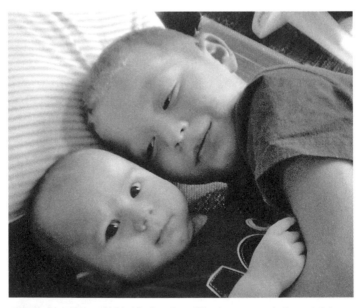

FIGURE 4.2. Alex and his big brother, Eli *(Photo courtesy of Amy Rohr)*

Brothers and sisters can be a big help when a child is in a cast or brace. They can bring toys to that child or pick up items that are dropped. Some families let older siblings decorate a plaster cast by drawing on it or coloring it (see Figure 4.3).

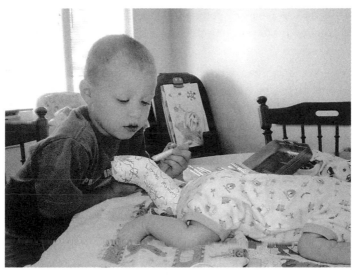

FIGURE 4.3. Eli decorating Alex's first cast *(Photo courtesy of Amy Rohr)*

Amy Rohr's younger son, Alex, was born with a left clubfoot. In the following passage, she describes how his older brother, Eli, reacted to the process of treating Alex's foot:

At [Alex's] birth, [the clubfoot] didn't seem to matter to Eli at all. In fact the whole process has been pretty easy for him to handle. In the beginning, we included him by letting him draw on and decorate Alex's casts, but that was when Alex stayed in one place. Once he was moved to braces, Eli was very sympathetic when he fussed as we put them on and such. He did ask lots of questions to clarify what exactly was wrong with [Alex's] foot, and we found that the easiest answer was to tell him that Alex's foot was a little crooked and that the doctor was going to straighten it out!

His biggest problems with the situation were:

- We had to drive three hours to our son's doctor and did this each week for a while. Since it was so long of a trip, we often left Eli with family. I think that was an additional shock to him when he was already getting used to not being the center of attention. A few of our trips we turned into mini vacations, and we stayed in motels, taking him along. That seemed to help.

- The other was the removal of casts and the doctor's messing with his brother. [Eli] was very overprotective and scared for Alex. I think he realized that Alex was too young to be scared for himself. The few times he has gone to an appointment with us he has stood by the exam table watching like a hawk. He would often ask if things hurt Alex or not. The biggest issue was the saw to remove the casts. The noise made Alex cry, and Eli thought that they were hurting him. Talk about chaotic!

[AMY ROHR]

Tovey has this to say about how her older children interacted with Jack when he was born with clubfoot:

Our kids were 14, 4, and 2 when Jack was born. The 14-year-old took everything in stride like an adult. His biggest concern was getting Jack's feet straight so he could play sports. Our 2- and 4-year-olds were oblivious to the concerns; I think mostly because my husband and I never acted like it was a big deal. We just told the little ones that God had made Jack with special feet and Dr. Ponseti was going to turn them into feet just like theirs. They loved the whole five weeks in Iowa and loved the clinic staff. During the casting phase, they would roll towels to put under Jack's knees and use wipes to clean his casts. They also loved to poke his toes to make sure they turned white then pink again.

After Jack got his shoes and brace it's been a daily fight [between the kids] to bring me the brace and help put on the shoes.

Now at [ages] 5 and 3, they know exactly how the shoes go on and love to click the shoes onto the brace, especially my 3-year-old. She could probably put the shoes and brace on Jack herself if he would hold still. They drag Jack everywhere in his brace, help him up and down the stairs and in and out of bed. They are also big helpers when Grandma and Grandpa or our baby-sitter has the kids and puts on the brace. They know exactly how the holes are supposed to be and my mother-in-law says that they say, "Tight, Nana. His shoes have to be tight!"   [TOVEY]

Have fun together and keep a positive attitude. Your children will take their cues from you. An illustrated children's story about clubfoot is included in this book. (See "Straight, Strong, and Stretchy: A Children's Clubfoot Story" on page 116.)

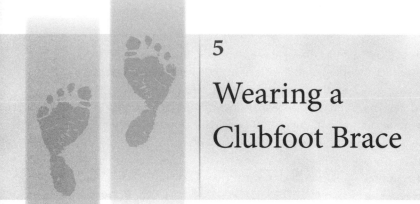

5

Wearing a
Clubfoot Brace

After your child's foot has been corrected, they wear a brace to keep the clubfoot from coming back. It is called a foot abduction brace (FAB). Examples of different types of FABs are shown in Figures 5.1, 5.2, and 5.3.

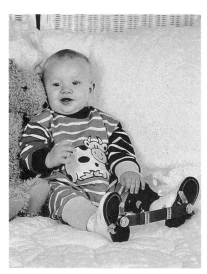

FIGURE 5.1. This baby is wearing an adjustable FAB with Markell shoes. *(Photo courtesy of Fillauer, Inc.)*

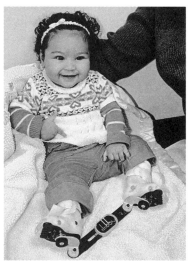

FIGURE 5.2. This baby is wearing a D-Bar FAB with custom AFOs. *(Photo courtesy of D-Bar Enterprises, Inc.)*

Note: A brace cannot correct clubfoot. If the child's foot is not corrected, the brace could be painful and the child's foot might slip out.

The brace consists of special shoes or ankle–foot orthoses (AFOs) with a connecting bar. An AFO can look like a shoe or sandal, but it must affect or control a joint—in this case, the ankle joint.

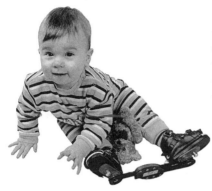

FIGURE 5.3. This baby is wearing an ALFA-Flex FAB with ALFA-Flex shoes. *(Photo courtesy of Semeda Medizinische Instrumente)*

Wearing the brace is required for successful treatment of clubfoot. Without a brace, the clubfoot is likely to come back. If this happens, the foot relapses and has to be corrected again. The following statistics show how crucial brace wear is to maintaining clubfoot correction:

- About 90 percent of babies who stopped wearing the brace as directed in the first year of treatment relapsed.

- For babies who stopped wearing the brace in the second year, 70 to 80 percent relapsed.

- In the third year, 30 to 40 percent of the babies who stopped wearing a brace relapsed.

As you can see, wearing the brace is an essential part of treatment for clubfoot. Most children with clubfoot must wear a brace at night until they are four or five years old. Research has shown what a difference wearing a brace makes. "A patient whose family does not comply with the protocol for the [clubfoot brace] is 183 times more likely to have a relapse than is one whose family complies."[1]

[1] Dobbs, M. B., J. R. Rudzki, D. B. Purcell, T. Walton, K. R. Porter, and C. A. Gurnett, "Factors Predictive of Outcome After Use of the Ponseti Method for the Treatment of Idiopathic Clubfeet," *Journal of Bone and Joint Surgery, Am* 86 (2004): 22–27.

Brace-wear Schedule

After your child's foot is corrected and the final cast comes off, your child starts wearing a brace right away. If the brace is not ready, the doctor applies a new cast to hold the foot in place so that it does not relapse while you are waiting for the brace. The age of the baby or child when the foot is corrected affects how many hours each day the brace must be worn.

- Young babies who are not yet crawling or walking wear the brace 23 hours per day for 3 months. Then the hours are gradually reduced month by month to 20 to 22 hours, 18 to 20 hours, 16 to 18 hours, and finally 14 to 16 hours. The child continues with the 14-hour schedule until age 4 or 5.

- Babies with feet that were corrected at around 8 or 9 months of age are ready for crawling and walking, so they do not wear the brace as many hours as the younger babies. Instead, they wear the brace 18 to 20 hours per day for 2 months, 16 hours per day for 3 or 4 months, and finally 12 to 14 hours per day until age 4 or 5.

- For older babies or toddlers with delayed treatment or relapsed feet, the doctor develops a brace-wear schedule based on the child's individual case of clubfoot. (See "Beginning Clubfoot Treatment with an Older Child" on page 44.)

When your baby or child first starts wearing the brace, your doctor will give you guidelines explaining how to work up to the required number of hours per day. Dr. Morcuende from the Ponseti Clubfoot Center explains how the brace-wear schedule developed:

> One of the problems [years ago] was that Dr. Ponseti recommended stopping the brace too early as we know now—[at the age of] one and a half or two years. That's why he had such a high number of relapses, but he treated up to 70 percent of them with ATT transfers.
>
> What happens now is a different story. Most use the brace up to the age of four or five. The number of relapses has decreased a lot, especially in the first few years. Most of the relapses are to do with

not wearing the brace in general. The rate of surgery now for re-lapses has decreased. In 2003–2004 only 2 or 3 percent of the kids required ATT transfer.[2] It was a huge difference.

[DR. JOSE MORCUENDE]

Your child should see the doctor again two weeks or a month after the first brace is fitted; then they should go back every three months until they are three years old. After that, follow-up checkups are either once or twice a year until the child is seven, and then every two years until they are grown.

Different Types of Braces

Some common braces are the Denis Browne bar, the Ponseti Club-foot brace, and the D-Bar brace. Most braces are designed to work with more than one kind of shoe or AFO. The following principles apply no matter which brace your child wears.

- Adjustable bars fit longer because they can be set wider as your child grows. You won't have to replace the brace as often.

- As your child outgrows shoes or AFOs, you can order larger sizes without replacing the bar.

- Shoes or AFOs with open toes and an open heel help you to see if your child's foot is completely inside.

- With quick-release style bars, the shoes snap on and off (see Figure 5.4). This makes it easier to put your child into a high chair or car seat.

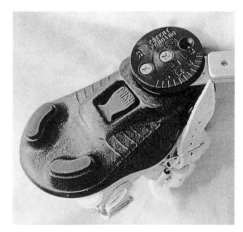

FIGURE 5.4. A quick-release Ponseti bar
(Photo courtesy of MD Orthopaedics, Inc.)

[2] Children who do not follow the brace-wear schedule are far more likely to need ATT transfer surgery.

Bars

Clubfoot braces include a bar that connects the AFOs or shoes that the child wears to hold their feet in the corrected position. Some settings vary a bit depending on the bar that is used. For example, a setting of 60 degrees of abduction (turnout) in the Ponseti–Mitchell brace (a Ponseti brace with Mitchell shoes) is equivalent to 70 degrees of abduction in the Denis Browne bar brace. A variety of bars are used to treat clubfoot. Some of the more common bars include the following:

- **Denis Browne bar (DBB).** This brace comes in a number of different styles. The adjustable, removable style fits the longest and is easiest to work with.

- **Ponseti clubfoot brace.** This brace was designed by Dr. Ponseti for clubfoot treatment. It is adjustable and can fit newborns up to three or four years old (see Figure 5.5).

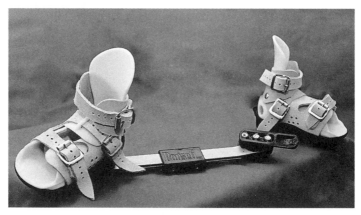

FIGURE 5.5. A Ponseti brace with Mitchell AFOs *(Photo courtesy of MD Orthopaedics, Inc.)*

- **D-Bar brace (Dobbs brace).** D-Bar braces (see Figure 5.6) also come in different styles. Some are made to work with specific AFOs or shoes. All are adjustable and can fit newborns and children up to four or five years old. D-Bar makes a dynamic bar that is hinged in the middle so that the child can move each foot independently.

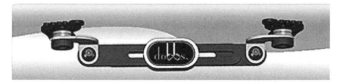

FIGURE 5.6. A D-Bar brace *(Photo courtesy of D-Bar Enterprises, Inc.)*

- **ALFA-Flex brace.** This brace is popular in Germany (see Figure 5.7). It is adjustable and has a click release.

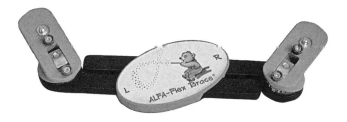

FIGURE 5.7. An ALFA-Flex brace *(Photo courtesy of Semeda Medzinische Instrumente)*

Shoes and AFOs

The shoes and AFOs are effective only when attached to the connecting bar. Wearing them without the bar does not work because they cannot hold the feet at the angle needed to maintain correction. Technically, any well-made shoes that hold the feet in a stable position could be attached to a bar to treat clubfoot if the feet are held at the correct angles. In the developing world a variety of shoes and bars are used.

Markell Shoes

Markell shoes (sometimes also called "boots") are straight last, which means that the left and right are the same shape. They are designed to work with the Denis Browne bar and many other braces. Markell shoes might not fit babies with atypical clubfoot if the heel cannot go down far enough into the shoe. The model with an open heel helps parents make sure that the baby's heel is all the way inside the shoe (see Figure 5.8 on the following page). For many children, the Markell shoes work just fine.

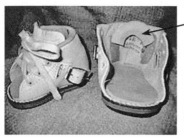

Neoprene shaped like an upside-down U was used to customize the fit of this shoe to help keep the foot from slipping.

FIGURE 5.8. Markell open-toed shoes *(Photo courtesy of Michael Colburn. DPM)*

Mitchell Shoes (AFOs)

Though they are AFOs, Mitchell shoes look like sandals (see Figure 5.9).

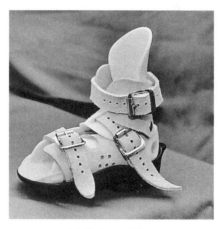

FIGURE 5.9. A Mitchell AFO *(Photo courtesy of MD Orthopaedics, Inc.)*

Mitchell shoes come in a wide range of sizes including very small sizes, such as 0000 and 000, which are suitable for premature babies. Mitchell AFOs are open-toed, and the back is open so that it is easy to see if the heel is completely in the shoe.

Note: The tongues on Mitchell shoes are long. You can tuck them in between the rubber and the leather. It is also okay to trim them if you want. Be sure to leave enough leather to protect your child's foot from pressure by the strap.

Mitchell Pressure Saddles

Pressure saddles reduce pressure from the brace to help the child's skin stay healthy while they are wearing the brace (see Figure 5.10). Some parents call these "Pringles" because of their shape.

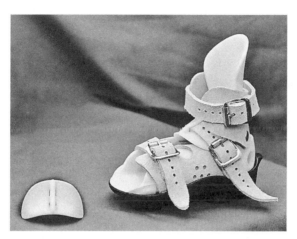

FIGURE 5.10. A pressure saddle with a Mitchell AFO
(Photos courtesy of MD Orthopaedics, Inc.)

Custom (Dobbs) AFOs

These open-toed AFOs have a soft fabric liner that fits inside shoes that are custom-made for your child (see Figure 5.11).

Before the custom AFOs are made, a certified orthotist makes casts of your child's feet. The first pair fits for about three months. These were designed by Dr. Dobbs, who also designed the D-Bar brace.

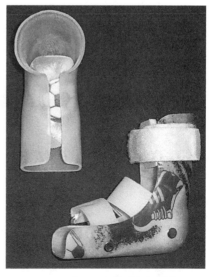

FIGURE 5.11. Custom (Dobbs) AFOs
(Photo courtesy of D-Bar Enterprises)

Other Shoes

The **ALFA-Flex shoes** shown in Figure 5.12 and the corresponding brace are popular in Germany.

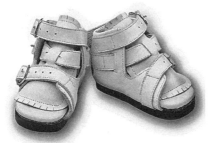

FIGURE 5.12. ALFA-Flex shoes *(Photo courtesy of Semeda Medizinische Instrumente)*

- **Plantarflexion stops.** These fit inside a shoe or AFO to keep the foot in a flexed position so that the heel stays down.
- **Plantarflexion stop sandals.** These sandals keep the foot in a flexed position so that it cannot point downward and the heel cannot come up.

Combining Bars and Shoes or AFOs

Most braces are designed to work with more than one type of shoe or AFO. Some combinations require adapters to attach the shoes or AFOs to the bar (see Figure 5.13).

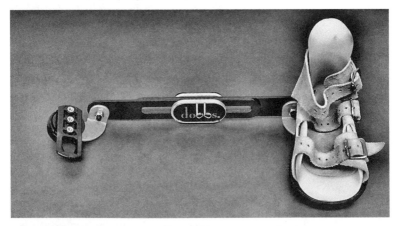

FIGURE 5.13. A D-Bar for Mitchell AFOs *(Photo courtesy of D-Bar Enterprises, Inc.)*

The doctor specifies in the prescription the type of brace your child will wear. Different doctors have preferences based on their experiences and your individual child's situation.

Ordering Your Child's First Brace

The doctor measures your child's feet and prescribes the brace at the visit when the final Ponseti cast is put on your child.

It is a good idea to contact your insurance company when your doctor prescribes the brace. Some insurance companies do not cover shoes even though the shoes are an essential part of the brace. In most cases, AFOs are covered. The brace usually is ordered through an orthotics facility. If the insurance company will not cover the brace, check to see if the office you are ordering the brace through is signed up to be a provider with your insurance company. If not, you might need to order the brace elsewhere to get coverage.

Ponseti braces and Mitchell AFOs are available through orthotics facilities or directly from MD Orthopaedics, Inc. If you plan to order directly, ask your doctor to call in the prescription to MD Orthopaedics or give it to you. Then contact MD Orthopaedics to place an order. This can be less expensive than going through an orthotics facility. As with all braces, a set of foot measurements is needed to make sure the brace and AFOs will be the right size. Usually the orthotist measures the feet, but if you order direct from MD Orthopaedics, you will need to measure your child's feet based on their instructions. Typically, the AFOS are a larger size than needed to allow for growth. If your child goes to an orthotics facility, a staff member will measure the feet. If you order directly from MD Orthopaedics, they will provide you with measuring instructions.

Fitting the Brace

Though a doctor and an assistant apply the serial casts, and the doctor prescribes the brace, they probably will not put the brace on your child. Usually an orthotist fits the brace. An orthotist is trained to make and adjust braces (orthoses). Some hospitals have Orthotics and Prosthetics (O & P) departments. There are also independent orthotic and prosthetic facilities. The orthotist measures your baby's or child's feet to make sure the brace will be the right size. If you order directly through MD Orthopaedics, they will ask you to provide measurements for your child's feet.

The orthotist uses the doctor's prescription as a starting point but will adjust the bar width to fit your child and position the angle of the shoes or AFOs.

To customize the brace fit for your child, the following guidelines are typically used:

- The bar between your child's heels should be a little wider than the width of their shoulders.

- The brace must hold the clubfoot at the correct angle to encourage the heel to stay down. This is 10 to 15 degrees of dorsiflexion. (See "Equinus, Dorsiflexion, and Plantarflexion" on page 18.) For some types of braces, the orthotist must add a bend to the bar or foot plates for this to occur.

- With a Ponseti bar, the clubfoot is rotated outward at 60 degrees. With a Denis Browne bar brace, the clubfoot is rotated outward at 70 degrees. If one foot is normal, it is rotated outward at 40 degrees.

- With Mitchell shoes when your child first moves up to a larger size, there might be extra room in the heel.

Special Considerations

- If a child has loose joints or hypermobility (joints that stretch farther than normal), the feet could be set to 30 to 40 degrees of abduction. This is to prevent the child from developing flat feet as a side effect of treatment.

- If the child has atypical (complex) clubfoot, the angle might be set to 40 degrees and then gradually increased to 60 degrees, which could take up to a year. Forcing the foot makes the brace painful and can hurt the child's foot. A child with atypical clubfoot might not be able to tolerate Markell shoes.

Checking the Fit of the Shoe at Home

Make sure that your child's heel is completely inside the shoe. If it isn't, the foot will be in the wrong position, and the shoe could irritate your child's skin.

1. Take the shoes off the brace. Remove the laces or open the straps and open the shoe.

2. Put the socks that your child wears with the brace on them, and then put the shoe on.

3. Check that the heel is flat against the back of the shoe. If it is, use a pen to mark a line where your baby's toes are in the front of the shoe. This is a guide to where your child's foot should be when wearing the shoe. When their feet grow, then you will need to make a new line.

Note: With Mitchell AFOs, the heel might not go down completely when your child first starts wearing a brace. It could take a few weeks for the heel to drop all the way down.

If your child's heel cannot go completely into the shoe, check with your orthotist or doctor to see if a there is a fit problem. If the shoe is the right size, the problem could be that the foot is not completely corrected or has relapsed. If that is the case, the foot must be corrected with serial casting before the child can wear the brace.

Getting Used to a Brace after Wearing Casts

Many children fuss for the first few days when they begin wearing a brace. They might have sore muscles or sensitive skin from the cast, and they could also be frustrated. With many types of clubfoot braces, your child must learn to move both legs together and at first might struggle to move them independently. To teach your child how to move and kick both legs at the same time, play with your child by gently pushing and pulling on the bar of the brace. Talk to your child or sing to them while doing this to make it fun.

To prevent bumps or bruises, it is a good idea to pad the bar in case it accidentally hits someone while your child is wearing the brace. Padding the bar can also protect your furniture. The Ponseti Clubfoot Center website suggests using a bicycle handlebar pad, or foam pipe insulation covered with fabric or tape.

It can take three to seven days for your baby to adjust when they first change from wearing casts to wearing a brace. Your child might need pain relief such as acetaminophen (Tylenol) or ibuprofen (Motrin) for the first few nights. This is due more to muscle aches from the cast than discomfort from the brace. When your child first goes from cast to brace, take off the shoes every three to six hours to check the skin. The one-hour out is best for a bath and bedtime routine. This helps the baby get used to putting on shoes at bedtime and will help with transition to nighttime-only wear.

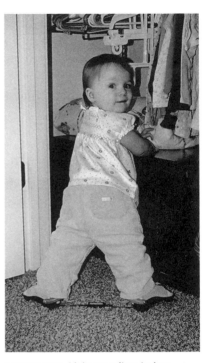

Children who are advanced enough in their development to stand or walk wear the brace for fewer hours than young babies. This helps them build muscle strength in their legs. As much as possible, try to schedule brace wear during nighttime. If your child stands or cruises in the brace (see Figure 5.14), that is fine.

FIGURE 5.14. Livie standing in her brace *(Photo courtesy of Debbie Monfort)*

Nicki's Reaction to Farley's Brace

Nicki's son Farley was diagnosed with clubfoot before birth during an ultrasound exam. In spite of Nicki's worries, Farley's serial casting went well. Still, Nicki was upset when she first found out about the brace that Farley had to wear. This quote describes her reaction and her experiences with Farley's brace wear over a four-year period:

When I saw those Ponseti–Mitchell shoes for the first time, I cried all over again. Four years of wearing these? You gotta be kidding me! They're torturous! Buckles and metal! How would he ever move around? How would he sleep? Twenty-three hours a day in these things? Would he ever learn to walk?

And yet, here we are, four years later, having complied with wearing those shoes every single night and nap—except on that flight to Sydney last year—we had to draw the line! The pipe insulation to keep him from killing his crib. The banging and kicking as he swung that thing around. Trying to get those things into a sling and figuring out how to breastfeed. The drudgery of having to explain them to babysitters and care providers. All those strange looks at playgrounds and airport security. The hot sticky humid nights when you couldn't believe you were putting socks and shoes on your child. The comedy of seeing your kid's foot resting high in the air as he slept. The panicked moments of returning back to the house to fetch them before we drove off again to preschool. The hundreds of dollars not covered by insurance. The removal for the third "Mama, I have to go potty" delay tactic of the evening. The triumph of being able to buckle those things in complete darkness. The loving care of the Mitchell family, who provided us about five different pairs over the years—the obvious commitment they have to this treatment. The PRIDE of knowing that all of this was an investment in a normal life.

[NICKI]

When confronted with your child's brace, don't panic. Ask questions if you are unsure about how to put it on or remove it. This does get easier with practice. The following sections in this chapter provide advice from experienced parents, orthotists, and doctors. If a problem arises that makes it hard for your child to wear the brace, get help. Work to solve the problem and follow the doctor's guidelines about how many hours per day your child must wear the brace.

Breastfeeding a Child in a Brace

Moms who breastfeed can continue while the child is wearing a brace. First, pad the bar in the brace to protect both you and the baby from bumps and bruises. Many mothers find it easiest to nurse in bed. Make sure that you are toward the middle of the bed so that you don't have to worry about your baby being too close to the edge. If you turn slightly to the side, this can make it easier for your baby to latch on. Prop a pillow below your baby's feet to support the brace and then position them for nursing.

Child Care

If your child is old enough to wear the brace only at nighttime, show the teacher how to remove the brace at a specific time such as noon or 10:00 AM. Using a removable bar makes it easier to put your child into a car seat. Remove the bar but leave the child's shoes on until they are strapped into the car seat. For a long drive, reattach the bar and repeat the process when you arrive at the day-care facility. For a short drive, you can leave the bar off until after you arrive.

Putting the Brace on Your Child

When your child is fitted with a brace, the orthotist shows you how to put it on your child. If you feel unsure, check to see if instructions came with your child's brace. There is a video at the MD Orthopaedics website that shows how to put on Mitchell AFOs. For young babies, you can practice taking off the brace and putting it back on while they are sleeping.

To start with, it might take two people to put on your child's shoes: one to distract them while the other puts them on. As you get more skilled at putting on the shoes and your child becomes used to it, this process goes more quickly. Some parents let their children watch a video while they put on the shoes. When your child changes to nighttime-only brace wear, make putting on the brace part of your bedtime routine. To put on the brace:

1. Put soft, 100 percent cotton socks on your child.
2. Take a minute to figure out which foot each shoe goes on. The straps fasten on the inside of the foot.
3. Put on the first shoe without the bar attached to it. Bend your child's knee to 90 degrees (at a right angle).

4. Fasten the laces or straps so that the shoe is snug.

5. Check the fit to make sure that the shoes are snug and the heel is all the way down inside the shoe.

6. Repeat steps 3 to 5 for the other shoe attached to the bar. Fasten the first shoe onto the bar.

Socks

Soft, thick socks that are 100 percent cotton seem to work best. Some parents cut out the toes, which makes it easy to check circulation. The shoes or AFOs should be tight enough to stay on, but the baby's toes should not turn purple or blue. If your child has sweaty feet, you might need to change the socks several times a day. Some socks that parents have been happy with are listed here:

- socks from The Children's Place
- Lamaze socks, available through Babies"R"Us or Toys"R"Us
- Gymboree-brand socks
- SmartKnit infant socks by Knit-Rite (These get mixed reports. Some parents like how well they wick moisture away from the foot, but others had problem with the socks bunching up.)
- Baby Hanes–brand socks

Your Child's Skin

Always check your child's skin when you remove the shoes. Swelling on the top of the foot is common with the Mitchell AFOs. This is harmless. It occurs because the middle strap does not allow the baby fat in that area to grow at the same rate as elsewhere. As your child outgrows baby fat, the appearance of swelling goes away. You might see red areas on your child's feet, but they should fade within about twenty minutes while the shoes are off. Skin problems to look for are blisters or pressure sores.

Red Marks with Mitchell Shoes

A red mark that doesn't go away twenty minutes after the shoe is removed can be a cause for concern.

- This can happen when a child is outgrowing shoes or when the flap is not flat as you tighten the strap.

- If the spot is in the center of the foot where the middle strap is, try loosening the middle strap. Pressure saddles can help too. (See "Mitchell Pressure Saddles" on page 71.)

- Make sure the single hole in the middle strap is above the buckle strap and make sure that it is tight. A loose strap could move and cause more irritation. If you are not sure how tight the strap is supposed to be, take your child to your doctor or orthotist and have them show you.

- If the problem continues, try moleskin or molefoam (available at drugstores) between the sock and the strap.

After you correct the problem, the red marks can take up to a week to clear up.

Bruising

If there have been some problems adjusting the shoes, your child might have bruises. Tovey describes how this happened to her son:

> It took Jack's bruise and redness about two weeks to go away completely. If the skin is not broken and if you lightly push on the redness and it goes away for a second, you are okay. The bruising goes away like any bruise in seven to ten days.   **[TOVEY]**

Blisters

Try to figure out where the shoe is rubbing the child's skin and adjust the fit. A wrinkle in a sock can cause a blister. Blisters can occur if the shoe is too loose and the child's foot slips up and down within the shoe. To prevent blisters from forming or getting worse, you can try the following ideas:

- Use molefoam or moleskin to protect a blister while it heals. The molefoam or moleskin goes between the sock and the shoe or AFO.

- Plastizote is a foam padding that can be used to customize the fit of your child's shoe or AFO, especially in the heel area.

- Thick socks sometimes help.

- Stretching exercises might help your child's foot go into the shoe more completely.

- If your child has blisters, try blister bandages from the first-aid section in drugstores. Carefully place the bandage over the blister.

If you are unsure about what to do, ask your child's orthotist or doctor for advice. If the blisters worsen, your child may not be able to wear the brace. Then the foot can relapse and need to be corrected again with serial casting. Have your child seen by or send a photo of your child's foot to the doctor to find out if the foot is not fully corrected. If the foot keeps slipping out of the shoe, that might be the reason.

If your child cannot wear the brace, talk to your doctor about a holding cast. Some children have a hard time tolerating Markell shoes. If this is the case, switching to Mitchell AFOs or custom AFOs may solve the problem. The orthotist also might be able to add a heel insert in the back of the Markell shoes.

Pressure Sores

A dark red area that does not fade when the shoe is removed can indicate a pressure sore that is forming. A pressure sore gets darker until it turns purple or black, and it can eventually become a painful open sore. A pressure sore is a serious skin problem that will not heal until the cause of the pressure is located and corrected. If you think one is developing, contact your orthotist or doctor immediately. If your child has a sore, they might need to stop wearing the brace until it heals. This does increase the risk of a relapse, so get your doctor's opinion about how to handle the situation. To help with pain relief, ask your pharmacist about a hydrocolloidal bandage. This is a special kind of bandage made for open sores or burns.

Wearing Shoes When the Brace Is Off

After your child starts to wear the brace only at night, they will need ordinary shoes to wear during the daytime. Bare feet are best, but for those times when shoes are needed, some families have had good luck with soft-soled shoes such as Robeez or New Balance athletic shoes (see Figure 5.15).

Have your child try on the shoes at the store before you buy them. If your child has different sized feet, you can try See Kai Run online or Nordstrom stores. (See "Socks, Shoes, and Sleep Sacks" on page 137 in the Resources section.)

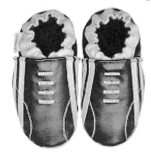

FIGURE 5.15. Robeez Soft Soles shoes *(Photo courtesy of Stride Rite)*

Helping Your Child Sleep with a Brace

Expect an adjustment period of up to three weeks while your child gets used to sleeping while wearing the brace. Many children are frustrated until they figure out how to move both feet simultaneously. If your child is old enough to roll over, they might need some time to figure out how to roll over in the brace. Babies do adjust and learn to sleep while wearing a brace, sometimes in unusual positions as you can see in Figure 5.16.

The following suggestions are from parents:

- Use pillows or rolled-up blankets to prop up your baby in a comfortable position. For example, when they are sleeping on their back, put a pillow under their knees.

- Some families use a breathable bumper such as the one from BreathableBaby available at Babies"R"Us. This protects the side of the crib.

- Children who are congested due to a cold or flu might sleep better in a car seat than a crib because their heads are elevated.

- If your child is old enough to sleep in a bed, consider putting a mattress on the floor. This makes it easier for a child to get into and out of bed while wearing a brace.

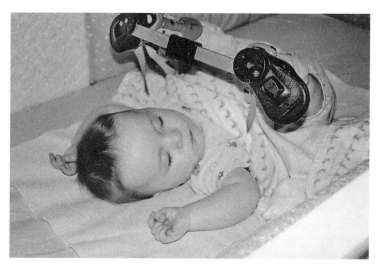

FIGURE 5.16. Livie sleeping in her brace *(Photo courtesy of Debbie Monfort)*

Based on the brace-wear schedule, your child will gradually change from full-time brace wear to wearing the brace from twelve to fourteen hours per night. It works best if the child wears the brace at night so that they can build muscle strength by moving during the daytime. Because children get used to being without the brace during the day, sometimes they resist going into the brace at nighttime even if putting on the brace has not been a problem in the past. It is best to create a bedtime routine that includes putting on the brace. For example, after bath time, the child could put on pajamas and the brace and then you could read a story together.

If your child is miserable, is sleeping poorly, and you don't know why, consider the following suggestions:

- Are they frustrated because they haven't learned how to roll over in the brace? Try helping them roll over until they learn this skill.

- If they had a recent growth spurt, they could be outgrowing the brace.

- If the brace gets tangled in the sheets and blankets, try using a sleep sack to keep your child warm without blankets. If the brace gets caught in the crib slats, you can cover the sides of the crib with a blanket. A portable playpen or crib with mesh sides might solve this problem.

- For some children, the brace bangs against the side of the crib or bed when they roll over. This might resolve on its own as your child gets used to rolling over while wearing the brace and figures out how much room is in the crib or bed. A portable playpen or crib with mesh sides might solve the problem, or consider putting your child to bed on a mattress on the floor.

Consider, also, that you might have a problem unrelated to clubfoot. Is your child learning to stand? Some toddlers who are reaching this milestone have trouble sleeping because they keep wanting to get up. This issue is unrelated to clubfoot, and the child will outgrow the problem. Check for teething and other common childhood issues that can interfere with sleep.

Outgrowing a Brace

If you notice an increased fussiness at night or that your child's toes curl completely over the front of open-toed shoes, it may mean that they are outgrowing the brace.

Adjusting the Bar

If your child has been sleeping fine in the brace and begins to have trouble at night, check to see if the bar needs to be wider. The bar should be the width of your child's shoulders or slightly wider. This is the most comfortable position for the child, and it changes as the child gets bigger. If you are handy, you can adjust the bar yourself; otherwise, take your child to the orthotist who fitted the brace. The Ponseti brace comes with an Allen wrench to loosen and tighten the bar when you make adjustments. Loosen the screws and adjust the bar to the right length (you can mark the proper length with a marker). Then tighten the screws.

New Shoes

Generally a baby needs two or three pairs of shoes the first year; after that they will need about one pair per year until age four or five. Custom AFOS that come with the D-Bar must be fitted by an orthotist, and they last about three months.

Some children's feet grow faster than others. The shoes need to fit in both the length and the width. If your child has a wide foot, they might outgrow the shoes even if there is enough room in the toe area. When your child gets a new, larger pair of shoes, it might take time to break them in. Some parents alternate nights between the old shoes and the new ones.

If you are replacing the shoes yourself (versus having an orthotist replace them), follow these steps:

1. Contact your doctor or orthotist and order a larger pair of shoes. Usually the next pair will be two sizes larger to allow for growth.

2. If the shoes have buckles, attach them with the buckles facing inside. Most shoes or AFOs click onto the bar.

3. Check the width of the bar. It should be the width of the outside of your child's shoulders. Widen it if necessary to account for your child's growth. It is okay to set the bar slightly wider if your child is more comfortable that way.

4. The first time your child wears the new shoes, mark a line to show where the toes are when the foot is completely inside the shoe. This line will change as your child grows. It can also change a few days after your child is out of a cast as the swelling goes down.

Tips for New Shoes

With a new pair of shoes, expect an adjustment period that can last from two to six weeks.

- Some parents alternate nights with the old shoes and the new shoes for a smoother transition.

- With a new pair of larger-size Mitchell AFOs, the heel pocket is deeper. It might take some time before your child's feet can stretch enough for the heels to move all the way down into the new AFOs.

- If you believe the new shoes are the wrong size, contact your doctor or orthotist. If you are able to email photos of your child's feet in the shoes, that might save you a trip.

- If you made adjustments to the old pair of shoes such as cutting a bigger slit for the strap in the tongue or adding padding, you might need to make the same adjustments to the new pair.

Donating Outgrown Braces

Your doctor or orthotist might be able to accept a donated brace or shoes if they are in good condition. Sometimes these items can be refurbished and made available to patients who might have difficulty affording new ones.

Solving Problems with the Brace

If you are struggling with your child's brace, don't hesitate to ask for help from your orthotist or doctor. Following the brace-wear schedule is the most effective way to prevent a relapse. Some common situations and suggestions that you can try are presented here.

Kicking Off the Shoes

Two main factors cause this:

1. The foot is not fully corrected.
2. The brace is not set up correctly. Check the width of the bar. Make sure that laces or straps on the shoes or AFOs are tight.

Your Child Removes the Shoes

If your child unfastens the straps or laces, you can try these tactics:

- For Markell shoes, reverse the laces, tie them at the bottom, and then use a double knot. Tighten the laces.
- Roll the top of the socks down to cover up the laces or straps.
- At night, use a sleep sack instead of pajamas.
- Use leg warmers such as those made by BabyLegs. Put them on so that they cover the buckles and straps.
- For Mitchell shoes, tighten the middle strap by one more hole. Remove the tongue of the shoe.

The Foot Slips out of the Shoe

Check the following:

- Is the foot still corrected or has it relapsed?
- Is the bar too narrow?
- Are the shoes fastened tightly so that the foot doesn't slip inside the shoe?
- Are the shoes too small?
- Use Velcro fasteners to help keep the sock inside the shoe. See the following section, "Tips from Parents."

Tips from Parents

Whether by wiggling out of shoes, or slamming their shoes down, some kids seem determined to get out of their shoes. Many families believe their babies have "little tiny Houdini feet" based on their ability to escape from shoes as well as the escape artist Harry Houdini might have done:

> Dino was actually a little legend in his own time on the nosurgery 4clubfoot site, because no matter what we tried, he escaped from his brace. He was nicknamed "Houdino" for his antics and kept us busy trying every little "fix" to keep him in those shoes. With all the back-and-forth messages between me and all the parents trying to help me with their own experiences, there's a wealth of info in the archives about how to keep those little feet in there.   [PAMELA]

The following suggestions come from parents of babies and children who are wearing clubfoot braces:

- Markell shoes might not be tight enough. If you are not sure how tight they should be, have your child's orthotist show you.
- For Mitchell shoes, fold down the top strap so that instead of sitting around the leg it sits just above the ankle. You can cinch this quite tight without the strap rubbing or causing pain.
- Put adhesive Velcro circles on the inside base of the shoe. Use two per shoe and attach matching Velcro to the bottom of the socks. Using this modification, one mom found that her

daughter could not get the sock out of shoe, though she did get her foot out of the sock once.

- An upside-down U of neoprene inside the back of the AFO or shoe might help keep the heel down. Neoprene is a synthetic rubber that is used in some clothing and shoes. Your orthotist or doctor can provide it.

Brace Maintenance and Repair

Mitchell shoes have a six-month warranty. If a strap breaks, you can contact MD Orthopaedics or bring the shoe back to the orthotics facility where your child was fitted. Then it can be repaired or replaced. If a warranty does not apply, you can also contact a cobbler or shoe repair business.

Some children manage to break the bar. If this happens, contact the place where you got the brace. For the Ponseti bar, there is a kit for the black plastic parts. If the metal bar breaks, it can be replaced. If this happens at night, you can try a temporary repair so that your child can continue to wear the brace. Some parents have used packing tape or duct tape. When Tovey's son Jack broke his brace, this is how she and her husband improvised:

> We snapped the black plastic piece that slides into the shoe. [To fix it for the night], we inserted a paint stirrer into the shoes and duct taped it to the brace. It held overnight, but it was a pain to peel off all the duct tape later. Necessity is the mother of invention they say.
>
> **[TOVEY]**

When Your Child Is Done with the Brace

While your child wears the brace, they go to the clubfoot doctor for exams. Most children wear a brace at night until age four or five. Eventually the day will come when the doctor tells you that your child no longer needs to wear a brace. Nicki describes this important milestone for her son Farley.

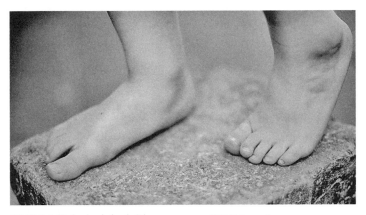

FIGURE 5.17. Farley's feet *(Photo courtesy of Nicki Dugan)*

I have been looking forward to this for four years. Not to gloat, but to encourage all of you who might be in the earliest stages of treating clubfoot and let you know that, yes, some day this will all be over!

This week, we got the brilliant news…Farley is officially 100 percent corrected! He has one helluva beautiful, gorgeous, and normal foot. We can finally retire our trusty Ponseti-Mitchells and enjoy the unbelievable novelty of sleeping in bare feet! And I can assure you that Farley runs, walks, hops, jumps, rides his bike, keeps up with his big brother, and NEVER complains. Yeah, he's going to have a slightly smaller calf when he hits puberty. But other than that, no one will ever know a thing about these last four years or how this little super hero stuck it out without so much as any pushback.

We are full of gratitude to Dr. Ignacio Ponseti, John Mitchell, Dr. Michael Colburn, and all of you [nosurgery4clubfoot members] for your wisdom, support, sharing, questions, answers, and reassurance. You go through so many stages: from clueless, anxious, and full of questions to a confident elder who has many answers and provides the comfort. Thank you, thank you. Keep doing what you do [in the nosurgery4clubfoot group]. It is the first place people discover when they get that diagnosis. Without you, this road would be dark, uncertain, and very lonely.   [Nicki]

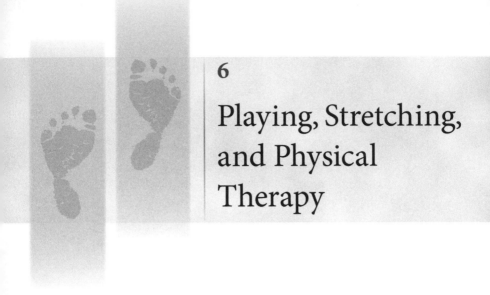

6

Playing, Stretching, and Physical Therapy

With clubfoot, the heel cord and the tendons and ligaments in the instep of the foot tend to be shorter and less flexible than usual. The clubfoot and calf also tend to have less muscle tone. As your child's foot is corrected, it becomes more flexible, though it probably will not be as flexible as a foot without clubfoot. Some clubfeet are stiffer than others, and each child's natural flexibility comes into play as well. If your child has only one clubfoot, you might notice that the clubfoot is less flexible than the other foot. This is typical, and it happens even with very successful clubfoot treatment. The most important thing is that the clubfoot has good alignment and is flexible enough for normal walking. Active play during the day when your child is out of the brace is a good way to build muscle tone.

The severity of clubfoot varies from one child to the next, and each child has their own unique natural level of muscle tone. Combine these considerations with different levels of physical activity and different growth rates among children, and it becomes clear that children undergoing the same treatment with a brace can end up with different levels of flexibility and muscle tone.

Play That Helps Your Child's Feet

The brace-wear schedule for your child takes into account the fact that it is healthy and fun for children to engage in active play. Because your child wears the brace at night, they are free to run around and play the same as any other child during the day.

Here are some fun activities that can help your child get stronger:

- Walking in sand helps stretch the Achilles tendon (heel cord).

- Pedaling a tricycle or bike builds muscle and keeps the feet flexed.

- When a child ice skates, the feet are in a flexed position.

- Using a trampoline or playing in a bouncy house builds both strength and flexibility.

- Active, imaginative play and dancing are also good for your child.

Stretching

Doctors vary in their approach to stretching and physical therapy after the foot is corrected. In the original Ponseti method, no stretches were included, but in the last several years, there has been a shift toward including stretches. The following sections describe two different approaches recommended by Ponseti-trained doctors, both of whom get excellent results with clubfoot treatment.

This is not to say that there might not be exceptions. Both doctors treat their patients individually and adjust treatment plans as needed based on each child's needs. Is active play enough to keep your child's foot and leg flexible and strong? The answer depends on the individual child and can change over time. When you take your child to see the doctor for a clubfoot exam, among other things, the doctor does check flexibility and strength.

The main benefits of stretching or physical therapy are increased flexibility, improved strength, and greater muscle tone. This can be especially helpful in keeping the tendons stretched when an older child is relapsing, which can occur during a sudden growth spurt if the Achilles tendon doesn't keep up with growth in the rest of the foot. In this situation, for some children stretching or physical therapy can make it less likely that the child will need a tenotomy (surgery to lengthen the Achilles tendon; see page 37) or ATTT surgery (tendon surgery to balance the foot; see page 102).

Method 1: Begin Stretches near the End of Brace Wear

To begin routine stretches near the end of brace wear is the more conservative approach of these two examples, and is typical of treatment at the University of Iowa Clubfoot Center. The original Ponseti method did not include stretching or physical therapy, but in recent years, as the original brace-wear schedule until age two has extended to age four or five, there has been movement toward adding stretches for children who are four or five years old (see Figure 6.1).

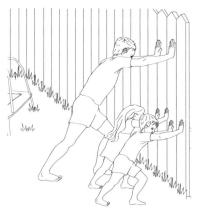

Doctors who use this method believe that for most children, active play is enough during brace wear. Unless there is a condition aside from clubfoot to address, no physical therapy or stretching is recommended until the child is around age four or five and is starting to transition out of wearing the brace.

In addition to stretching, use of a trampoline is recommended to help keep the Achilles tendon flexible (see Figure 6.2).

FIGURE 6.1. Dr. Morcuende often recommends a runner's stretch to flex the foot.

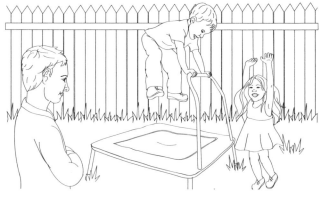

FIGURE 6.2. Using a trampoline can help keep the Achilles tendon flexible.

Dr. Jose Morcuende from the Ponseti Clubfoot Center explains how the role of physical therapy together with the Ponseti method has evolved over the years:

> When Dr. Ponseti practiced many years ago, he didn't use physical therapy at all as a complement of the treatment.
>
> If you do stretching exercises and try to keep the Achilles tendon (heel cord) stretched as much as you can during that transition from brace wear to no brace wear, the hypothesis is that you won't need that many ATT transfer [surgeries] to prevent relapses. That's why physical therapy is coming up, especially in the transition between brace and no brace.
>
> The stretches are for the heel cord, similar to what most runners do. These are simple stretches and [we also recommend] the use of a trampoline. We don't have data yet to show that this is making a difference. We started about a year and a half ago [in 2008]. We are putting together the data, waiting a bit for the follow-up. Hopefully within the next year and a half we will have some data on these patients to see what happens. It looks like it's working, but there aren't any [medical] papers [published] yet.
>
> **[DR. JOSE MORCUENDE]**

Method 2: Stretch the Child's Feet Throughout Brace Wear

Other doctors recommend performing stretching exercises throughout the brace-wear period. Doctors who use this approach see stretching as a noninvasive way to improve flexibility and strength in a child's foot. Many families find that during brace wear their children enjoy stretching, and it helps keep their child's feet flexible. Dr. Matthew Dobbs recommends this approach. He and his nurse teach parents exercises to help stretch their children's feet.

The following sections show stretching exercises that can be done while a child is out of the brace. If you are interested in the stretches, but unsure about using them, ask your child's doctor or a physical therapist to show you how to do them.

Ankle Stretch

This stretch is also called ankle inversion and eversion.

1. Lay your child on their back. Use one hand to hold the leg steady. With the other hand, grasp the outside of the foot.

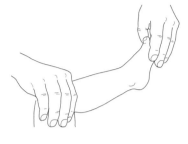

2. Gently turn the foot outward.

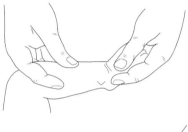

3. Then gently turn the foot inward.

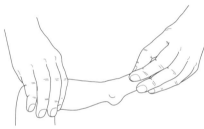

Heel Stretch

When your baby's brace-wear hours have been reduced to naps and nighttime, you can use these stretches to help keep the Achilles tendon (heel cord) flexible.

1. Lay your child on their back. Use one hand to hold the leg steady. Place the other hand on the bottom of the foot.

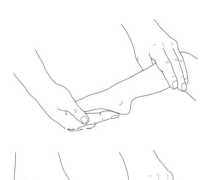

2. Push up on the front of the foot so that the heel comes down. Without hurting your child, bend the ankle as much as possible.

Seeing a Physical Therapist

If your child is age three or younger and needs physical therapy, they will most likely be referred to early intervention services (see "Early Intervention Services" on page 26). If your child is entering a physical therapy program, it could take six to eight weeks for you to notice improvement in flexibility and strength. Some of the most used physical therapy movements are listed here.

- stretching to improve flexibility
- walking up and down a ladder or walking up and down stairs
- hopping on one foot and then hopping on the other foot

Some other exercises are done while sitting. When sitting on a chair with foot and heel on the floor, the child tries to turn the foot outward to touch an object and then brings the foot back to a straight position. With the heel on the floor, the child taps the foot (raising the toes and putting them back down).

Early Intervention Services

The federal Individuals with Disabilities Education Act (IDEA) requires states to provide early-intervention services to eligible children and families. Children with clubfoot who need physical therapy typically qualify for these services. Each state has a separate organization, so you need to contact the one for your location. Sometimes there is a delay of a few weeks before your child can be seen by a physical therapist, but an early intervention staff person does need to see your child within forty-five days from the referral date. This is a federal mandate that all states must follow. If you are worried about the wait, ask your doctor to recommend stretches that you can do until your child is seen.

The physical therapist assesses the child and recommends therapy. If your state's early-intervention provider cannot deliver the services that your child needs, the staff will refer you to a facility where your child can receive the treatment that they need.

Stretching the Toes

In some children with clubfeet, their small toes tend to move together rather than separately. Some physical therapists recommend daily massages to stretch the toes out in this situation. You can do this after bath time before bed. Stretching at this time is good because the warm bath water can make the ligaments easier to stretch.

To stretch your child's toes to improve flexibility, try this process:

1. Put one hand in the front and one on the back of the toes and upper foot.

2. Start at the ball of the foot below the toe and work your way to the joints between the toes. Continue to the top of the toes.

3. Pull and work each toe individually to make sure that it can move separately. Use a firm but gentle touch so that you do not hurt the child. This should not hurt.

You will feel the toes loosen up and become more flexible as you do this.

Infant Massage (Not Part of Treatment)

Though massage is not part of clubfoot treatment, some babies like to have their feet and legs massaged when they are out of the brace. This section is for families who would like to explore this option.

When your baby is wearing the brace, especially during full-time wear (twenty-three hours per day), their feet and legs can become sensitized to the brace. This means that when the cast or brace is removed, their feet are tender to the touch. If this happens, massaging their feet and legs could help them feel better. This section offers some techniques that you can use to massage your baby's feet and legs. And if you want information beyond what is presented here, many books and websites cover the topic of infant massage. The important point to remember: When massaging your baby, look for cues that they enjoy the massage. If your child does not like being massaged, stop and do not force the issue.

To massage your baby:

1. Massage one leg at a time. While your child is lying down, stroke their leg gently from the knee to the foot. Then stroke in the opposite direction from the ankle up to the hip.

2. Use your thumbs to massage the bottom of the foot and the top of the foot from toes to ankle.

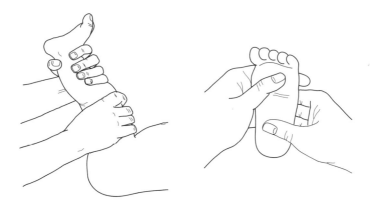

What Is French Physical Therapy?

The French physical therapy program is not associated with the Ponseti method, though its goals are the same. With the French method, physical therapy, taping, and splints are used to correct clubfoot and hold it in the corrected position until age two. Parents must learn stretching techniques for their children during treatment. The French physical therapy method includes these steps:

1. **Physical therapy.** A physical therapist stretches and massages the baby's foot daily and tapes the foot to hold it in place.

2. **Parent participation.** The physical therapist teaches parents the techniques to work with the baby's foot. Parents work with their baby to do the daily stretches and taping for eight to twelve weeks.

3. **Achilles (heel-cord) tenotomy.** The majority of children need a tenotomy so that the heel can move downward.

4. **Splinting.** Older babies and toddlers wear splints to hold the foot in place. The child wears the splints until age two.

Studies have shown there is an increased risk of relapse when clubfoot treatment is stopped at age two. The French method is not widely practiced in the United States, though Texas Scottish Rite Hospital for Children has a French physical therapy program. For more information, see the Resources chapter.

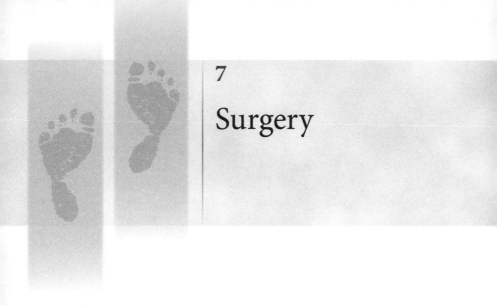

7
Surgery

With current methods of clubfoot treatment, most babies and children do not need surgery beyond a percutaneous tenotomy to release the Achilles tendon. (See "Lengthening the Achilles Tendon [Percutaneous Achilles Tenotomy]" on page 37.) In some cases additional surgeries are needed to correct more complicated cases of clubfoot. A Ponseti-trained doctor will correct the foot as much as possible with stretching and casts before any surgeries are considered. This approach results in less-invasive surgeries than the ones that doctors used before the Ponseti method was developed. The most common concern associated with foot surgery is scarring that can lead to less flexibility in the foot over the long term.

Preparing for Surgery in a Hospital

If your child will be admitted to a hospital, the doctor or hospital staff provides instructions about how to prepare your child for surgery. If general anesthesia will be used, your child probably will not be allowed to eat for at least eight prior to the surgery. Many doctors consider breast milk to be a clear liquid, which is allowed to be consumed up to four hours before surgery even if the child cannot eat food.

- Find out if your child can be scheduled for surgery early in the day. This can make it easier to manage withholding food.

- Ask if you can speak with another parent whose child has undergone similar surgery for clubfoot. You can also get in touch with other parents through support groups such as the nosurgery4 clubfoot online group. See "Clubfoot Information and Support Groups" in the Resources chapter.

Talking to an Older Child

It is best to tell an older child (those ages two and up) that they are going to have surgery. Use simple language that the child can understand. Explain that you want them to have the surgery to help their foot. Assure them that you will be nearby in the hospital while the surgery is taking place and during their recovery.

Your child might like to make a cast for a doll or stuffed bear at home before they go to the hospital. Some hospitals have programs through which the child can visit the facility to get used to the setting before the day of surgery. Children are shown a hospital gown, gas mask, and other equipment. If your child is much older (six years and up), take some time to explain the surgery to them or ask the doctor to explain it to them while you are present.

Taking Time Off

In the United States, depending on the size of the company for which you work, the Family and Medical Leave Act (FMLA) might allow you to take up to twelve weeks unpaid leave per year to care for a family member. This is the same act that covers maternity leave, and it can be helpful if a child needs surgery. If your child is already attending day care, they can continue going during treatment after recovering from surgery. (See "Child Care" on page 59.)

What to Bring to the Hospital

If you need to bring a diaper bag with you on the day of your child's surgery, put the most important items in the diaper bag. If your child will be staying overnight, pack a second, larger bag. Leave the larger bag in the car until after the surgery. When you have a room, retrieve the bag from the car or ask someone to bring it to you. The following sections offer suggestions about what to bring with you when you go to the hospital.

In the Diaper Bag

These items should fit into most diaper bags:

- your child's favorite blanket or stuffed animal
- extra pacifiers if your child uses them
- snacks such as crackers and juice boxes or a sippy cup for your child
- diapering supplies

In Your Purse or Wallet

These items are helpful in getting through the hospital paperwork and passing the time while your child is in surgery:

- your photo ID
- a folder with insurance cards, referrals, and medical information
- a cellular (mobile) phone or change for a pay phone, along with a list of phone numbers of friends and family to call after the surgery
- snacks or change for vending machines
- a book, magazine, or deck of cards

For an Overnight Stay

If your child needs surgery that will require them to stay overnight, bring these items:

- Your child's clothing. Bring socks, a shirt, pajama top or nightgown, and shoes (if your child wears them).
- New books or toys for your child. If you have a portable DVD player, bring it along with some favorite movies. You might also consider special items your child might enjoy, such as a balloon from the hospital gift shop, to keep them amused and make them feel special.
- If you are staying overnight, bring comfortable clothes for yourself. Sweats work well for nighttime. Also bring a towel, slippers, a book, magazine, or laptop computer, and snacks. If you are breastfeeding, consider bringing a breast pump.
- Some parents bring a box of candy for the nurses and staff members. If you want to take pictures, bring your camera.

Anesthesia

Before some types of surgery, a child is given general anesthesia to provide pain relief and to put them to sleep. Your child could be given either gas or an IV, and might also have an epidural (see "Epidural" on page 102). A pediatric anesthesiologist usually handles pain relief when a child has surgery. These doctors have special training to work with babies and children. Some hospitals allow a parent to take the child into the operating room.

If an older child is nervous and scared about the surgery, they could be given a "cocktail" such as liquid diazepam (Valium) to calm them down first. For a longer procedure, children two years of age or older might also be given some medicine to prevent nausea and vomiting during recovery. Usually these medicines are not needed for younger babies. Young babies are less likely to be scared or to experience nausea or vomiting after surgery. If your child is under two years old and has had nausea or vomiting after anesthesia in the past, tell the doctor, and ask for medicine to help keep it from happening again.

Note: Usually the cocktail and antinausea medicines are not given before very short procedures, such as a percutaneous tenotomy. This is because the effects can last longer than the procedure. If the child is still groggy from the "cocktail," it can complicate recovery.

If you are able to meet the pediatric anesthesiologist before surgery, ask the questions listed below:

- How long have you practiced?
- How will you put my child to sleep (with gas or a needle in the arm with medicine)?
- How long will it take before the drug is out of my child's system? Will my child be cranky? Will they recognize me?
- Can my child take a favorite toy into the operating room for comfort?
- What kind of side effects can we expect with the anesthesia?
- Will you be present for the entire procedure, or will someone else take over once the initial anesthesia is given?

Epidural

For some surgeries, an epidural is used in addition to general anesthesia. An epidural is pain medicine that numbs and blocks pain and is given through a soft tube, called a catheter, into the epidural space. The epidural space is near the backbone and spinal cord. The pediatric anesthesiologist uses a needle to insert the epidural and then tapes the tube so that it stays in place during surgery. The medicine comes from an epidural pump on a pole near the bed. With the epidural, a smaller dose of pain relief medicine can be used for just the right area of your child's body. A smaller dose of medicine can reduce side effects because less general anesthesia is needed. Sometimes the anesthesiologist places the epidural before surgery while the child is in the operating room (OR).

Note: With an epidural there is the chance that it will not provide complete pain relief (some women have this problem during childbirth). The pediatric anesthesiologist can adjust the pain-relief medicine if this happens.

An epidural provides pain relief for several hours after surgery and can let the muscles relax, which reduces muscle spasms. For a surgery in which the child will remain in the hospital overnight, the epidural might be left in place until the child can tolerate oral pain medicine. When your child can eat and drink, typically they are given medicine orally (by mouth), and the IV or epidural medication is stopped. Often the pediatric anesthesiologist continues to be involved after the surgery to help with pain management. Ask if this is the case at your hospital.

Balancing the Ligaments in the Foot with ATTT

ATTT (anterior tibialis tendon transfer) surgery is sometimes required to maintain the clubfoot correction in older children if the child's foot continues to relapse when the child is wearing a brace. This can be associated with neuromuscular clubfoot. Typically doctors wait until a bone in the foot called the lateral cuneiform has ossified (become solid), usually around thirty months of age.

Before ATTT surgery, the doctor corrects the foot as much as possible with the Ponseti method, and the child might participate in physical therapy. The purpose of ATTT surgery is to correct an imbalance in tendons in the foot that is causing heel varus (see "Varus and Valgus" on page 21) and supination (see "Supination" on page 20). In this situation, the tendons on the inside of the foot are stronger and tighter than the tendons on the outside of the foot. So the doctor moves the anterior tibialis tendon to the outside of the foot. A button on the sole of the foot holds the stitches that anchor the tendon in its new position. A cast is applied to hold the foot in position.

Usually an Achilles tenotomy is also needed to release the heel so that it can drop down. When a doctor corrects a clubfoot, the heel is the last part of the foot that is corrected, so these surgeries might be done together.

The child is put to sleep with general anesthesia for this procedure, and local anesthesia is also used. Usually the child stays overnight at the hospital and leaves with a long-leg cast, which is worn for about six weeks after surgery. Some children need physical therapy after the cast is removed to help their muscles get stronger and to improve their gait.

How the Doctor Performs ATTT Surgery

Here are the main steps involved in ATTT surgery:

1. Your child is given anesthesia.
2. The doctor performs the surgery and sews up the incision with dissolvable stitches. A button on the sole of the foot anchors the stitches. It is similar to buttons used on clothing.
3. The affected leg is put in a cast to hold the foot in position.
4. Your child is moved to the recovery room, where they are monitored and given pain relief medicine as needed.
5. The cast is worn for five or six weeks.

Your doctor will advise you as to how long your child should wait before standing or walking. A pediatric wheelchair can be useful for an older child. To keep your child occupied, consider using videos and books from the library, building toys such as Lego, and other games and activities that can be done while sitting.

Amelia's ATTT Surgery

Amelia's clubfoot was not treated until she was adopted at sixteen months of age. In addition to clubfoot, she has some nerve damage in one leg and has developmental dysplasia of the hip (DDH). The nerve damage affected Amelia's treatment for clubfoot. After her feet were corrected, one foot relapsed even though she had been wearing a brace as directed. Her mother, Kim, describes Amelia's ATTT surgery at age two years and seven months. Dr. Dobbs performed this surgery.

Amelia had two weeks of serial casting before the ATTT surgery. The surgery didn't take too long—about two hours. She spent one night in the hospital and was then released. Her pain was managed very well with liquid oxycodone and ibuprofen. We made sure that she got it every four hours as prescribed for a couple of days after we returned home, and then we started to stretch out the times and weaned her off completely after being home four or five days (I think—I know it wasn't long). We put ice packs on her legs to help with swelling, and it did help a great deal. We kept her legs elevated for a couple of days after the surgery also. After the surgery, she was in a first set of casts for two weeks.

Amelia was able to crawl around when she was pain free. She dragged herself all over the place just like she did when she was wearing her other casts. The biggest problem was that this particular set of casts was not covered in the fiberglass. Dr. Dobbs split the cast to help with swelling and then they wrapped the casts with ace bandages. Needless to say, she trashed them. We would remove the bandages to wash them and put clean ones on. It really wasn't a big deal though. The only other problem we encountered was that Amelia did "smash" the cast a little too much. She would lift her heel and then drop it on the floor and the heel of the cast was pretty much gone! She had to have a new cast put on because of that and getting the cast wet from playing in water—oops!

When we returned to St. Louis for the fiberglass overwrap, the cast was replaced because of some water damage and pretty bad wear and tear that I allowed (crawling on the driveway and so on). She was recast and still not permitted to bear weight for the remaining two weeks. At four weeks post op, the cast and button on the bottom of her foot were removed.[1] She was then put in short-legged casts for two weeks. During this time, she was allowed to bear weight and, believe me, she was doing it almost immediately. Two weeks later, the short-legged casts were removed, and she was put into a special "boot" that was for support. She was supposed to wear the boot for a couple of weeks since most kids won't walk for about that amount of time after the button and final casts are removed. Amelia chucked the boots after a couple of days and was back in her regular shoes walking, much to everyone's surprise.

[KIM]

Z-Lengthening Achilles Tenotomy

This surgery is more invasive than a percutaneous tenotomy. It is sometimes used for children aged three or older to release the heel if other techniques have not worked. When the heel drops down, the sole of the foot can be placed flat on the floor and the foot can flex upward. (See "Equinus, Dorsiflexion, and Plantarflexion" on page 18.)

The child is put to sleep with anesthesia. During the z-lengthening the doctor makes three cuts, each of which goes part-way through the Achilles tendon. The "Z" refers to the angle of the cuts. This can leave a scar about 1-inch long over the Achilles tendon.

How the Doctor Does the Z-Lengthening

The doctor's office or hospital provides instructions about how to prepare your child for this surgery. The doctor performs the z-lengthening procedure like this:

1. The child is given anesthesia.

2. The doctor makes three cuts in the Achilles tendon.

3. To lengthen the Achilles tendon, the front of the foot is stretched upward.

[1] The button anchors the stitches in place while the foot heels.

4. The doctor put stitches in the tendon and in the skin to close the incision. Typically the stitches are dissolvable and will not need to be removed later.
5. A cast is put on the foot to hold it in place.
6. The child is moved to the recovery room and monitored until they wake up.

Your doctor will advise you about pain relief for your child during the first day or two after the tenotomy. You will be given instructions for managing your child in a cast. The child wears a cast for at least three or four weeks, and, in some cases, up to six weeks. At first the child wears a long-leg cast, but for the final two weeks, a short-leg cast might be used.

Additional Surgeries

In some cases, other surgeries are needed.

Releasing a Big Toe Tendon (Great Toe Flexor Percutaneous Tenotomy)

Some children with atypical clubfoot have a big toe that sticks up and will not lie flat. If it does not correct itself, the doctor can surgically release it. This is a quick procedure. During the surgery a small cut is made on the bottom of the foot. This might be done at the same time as an Achilles tenotomy.

Posterior Tibial Tendon Transfer for Neuromuscular Clubfoot

Most children with clubfoot do not need posterior tibial tendon transfer (PTTT) surgery. PTTT surgery is associated with nerve damage or cerebral palsy (CP) that has occurred together with the clubfoot. If it is thought that a child with clubfoot has a nerve problem, the pediatric orthopedic doctor examines the child and might perform a nerve conduction test or an electromyogram (EMG). The outcome of these tests affects how the doctor treats the child. Some children wear a hinged AFO during the daytime and a clubfoot brace at night. The goal of PTTT surgery is to use the parts of the foot that are working to help the parts that are not. If this surgery is needed, it is usually performed on older children, not babies or toddlers.

Recovery from Surgery

Your child will probably be able to come home right after a percutaneous Achilles tenotomy. If general anesthesia is used or your child has additional surgery, they might stay overnight. During this time, pain medicine is often needed. Your child's doctor will write instructions on your child's chart for pain relief. This can avoid delays if medicine is needed when the anesthesia wears off. If your doctor gives you a prescription, fill it at the hospital pharmacy if possible. You can avoid a possible delay in case your local pharmacy doesn't have the medicine.

For a surgery in which the child remains in the hospital overnight, an epidural might be left in place until the child can tolerate oral pain medicine. Other times the anesthesiologist or surgeon orders pain medication on a pump, especially if the child is older. The child presses a button to get more medicine as needed. This is called a patient-controlled anesthesia (PCA). When your child can eat and drink, typically they are given medicine orally, and the IV or epidural medication is stopped. For information about pain management at home, see "Pain Management after Surgery" on the next page.

Take whatever supplies the nurses give you, such as moleskin and tape. Even if you can't use them right away, they will come in handy later when you are at home. It is a good idea to change your child's diaper before you leave the hospital. This gives you a chance to manage a diaper change where support is available if you need it. This also can prevent the child's diaper from leaking into the cast on the way home.

Tip: After surgery, your child might be given a device called an incentive spirometer to help clear out their chest from the anesthesia. This expands the lungs to prevent pneumonia. If your child hesitates, does not know what to do, or is afraid, ask about using a familiar toy such as a pinwheel or bubbles instead. For example, if a child can blow ten bubbles an hour, that works as well as the incentive spirometer.

Swelling

Swelling is common after surgery. Your child's cast might be tight for a few days until the swelling goes down. Ice packs can help reduce swelling and alleviate pain.

Muscle Spasms

During the first few days after surgery, your child might have muscle spasms. If a child has muscle spasms, pain medicine such as acetaminophen with codeine (Tylenol with codeine) or diazepam (Valium) is given to treat the spasms. Pain medicine might also be needed, but if the spasms are controlled, this decreases pain. Moving the child's feet during the day can help minimize spasms.

Scars

Scarring depends on the child's skin type and the kind of surgery. If you are concerned about scars, ask the pediatric orthopedic surgeon if it is possible for a plastic surgeon to close the incision to minimize scarring.

Eating after General Anesthesia

Some children have trouble with constipation after surgery. When a child is constipated, they have hard stools that could be painful for them to pass. If this happens, check with your pediatrician's office for suggestions about how to reduce the constipation. Some common drinks and foods that can help your child be more regular are fruits, fruit juices, vegetables, and whole grains. Other foods, such as rice, can contribute to constipation. Your pediatrician's office should have a list of foods that help a child who is constipated and foods to avoid. Many parenting books also include this information. Some children find it easier to have a bowel movement when they are lying on their stomachs.

Pain Management after Surgery

Some prescription pain relievers for children are acetaminophen with codeine (Tylenol with codeine) and hydrocodone with acetaminophen (Vicodin, Anexsia, Lorcet, or Norco). These medications can work very well to relieve pain, but since they are opiates, they also can make the child sleepy and constipated. Make sure that you keep all medicines out of reach of children, and throw away any remaining medication after your child is better. These drugs can be dangerous if overused. Your pharmacist can give you instructions for safe disposal of medication. Guidelines are also available on the website for the Institute for Safe Medication Practices at www.ismp.org (search for "throw away medicine").

If your child is taking acetaminophen with codeine and is not getting enough pain relief, notify your doctor. About 10 percent of people do not metabolize codeine effectively because their bodies do not break it down into the substances that relieve pain. If this is the case for your child, the doctor can prescribe a different medicine. If stronger pain relief is needed, such as after a more complex surgery, the doctor might prescribe a medicine such as oxycodone (Oxydose) for the child. If the child is very anxious, then lorazepam (Ativan) might be prescribed at bedtime to help them sleep.

How much pain medicine a baby or child needs depends on their weight. Make sure that you have a medication made for your child's size. If you have a baby, use infant medication. This is safer for the baby and protects against overdosing. Read the label carefully and if you have any questions, ask a pharmacist. They are trained to explain medication and can help you dose your child correctly. Once you locate the right dose, you must measure it accurately. A household teaspoon might not be accurate. Check with your pharmacist about the best device for measuring liquid medicines.

After surgery, your child's pain should decrease each day. If there is a sudden increase in pain and you do not know why, contact your doctor's office for advice.

Surgical Procedures Not Associated with the Ponseti Method

This section gives a brief description of surgeries that are not typically used by Ponseti-trained doctors.

Botulinum Toxin Injection for a Relapsed Clubfoot

Using botulinum toxin (BTX) injections to treat clubfoot is relatively new and has limited applications. BTX has been associated with some side effects, so make sure you understand possible risks before considering this procedure.

BTX is similar to Botox. BTX relaxes muscles, but it does not relax tendons or ligaments. Usually in clubfoot, the tendons and ligaments play more of a role in the foot alignment problems than the muscles do. If the tendons and ligaments have already been stretched and there is a residual muscle imbalance, then BTX could be helpful. Children with neurological disorders are unlikely to benefit from BTX.

Posterior Release or Posteromedial Release

Posterior release, or posteromedial release (PMR), surgery involves extensive changes to the foot and usually results in long-term stiffness as a side effect. PMR surgery used to be common before the Ponseti method was widely adopted. Today it is a last resort that is rarely needed to correct a clubfoot. If a doctor recommends PMR for your child, get a second opinion from a well-established clubfoot center with doctors who are highly skilled in the Ponseti method. It is best to correct the foot without surgery or with as few surgeries as possible.

Children who have undergone PMR surgery and still have clubfeet that are not fully corrected or have relapsed may still benefit from the Ponseti method. The Ponseti Clubfoot Center can provide advice in this situation.

The purpose of PMR surgery is to lengthen the Achilles tendon, but instead of cutting only the tendon, the doctor opens up the back of the foot. The surgery might involve releasing the ankle and subtalar joints. It is like taking apart the back of the foot and reconstructing it. This surgery can result in a stiff foot with a limited range of motion.

Surgery for Adults with Arthritis
Due to Clubfoot

Adults who were treated for clubfoot during infancy or childhood with the Ponseti method typically do well. Those who underwent extensive surgical procedures tend to do less well due to scarring and stiffness in the foot. This can lead to arthritis just as having clubfeet that were not completely corrected can.

The Ponseti method is not used for adults because their bone structure is already established. Adults with a clubfoot problem should see a podiatrist who is experienced in treating clubfoot. If the arthritis is severe, the doctor might recommend triple arthrodesis surgery. This surgery is used to treat severe, disabling arthritis in joints for which a joint replacement would not work, such as the ankles, wrists, thumbs, or toes. Arthrodesis is sometimes needed for adults who have clubfeet that were not completely corrected or were left untreated.

The purpose of this surgery is to relieve chronic pain and mobility problems in the foot and to improve alignment. Seek out a podiatrist experienced in this treatment who is knowledgeable about clubfoot. During surgery, the doctor fuses these three joints in the back of the foot:

1. subtalar joint (STJ)

2. talonavicular joint (TN joint)

3. calcaneal-cuboid joint (CC joint)

The patient wears a cast while the foot heals, followed by a medical boot when they first start bearing weight. Physical therapy might be needed to regain muscle strength and to improve flexibility.

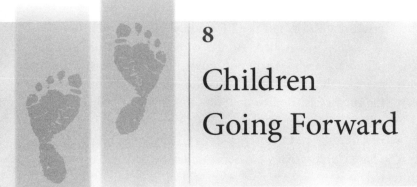

8

Children Going Forward

This book describes clubfoot and how the Ponseti method can treat this condition. Take some time to remember that what is really important are the children who benefit from the study and treatment of this condition.

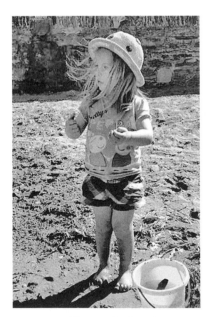

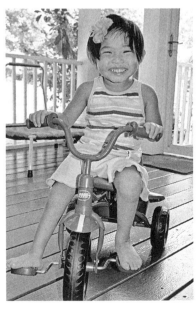

FIGURE 8.1. Fleur at the beach *(Photo courtesy of Erwan Creteur)*

FIGURE 8.2. Lia on her tricycle *(Photo courtesy of Kristen Trangsrud)*

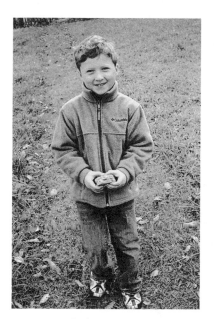

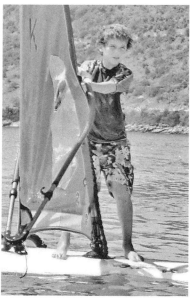

FIGURE 8.3. Farley *(Photo courtesy of Nicki Dugan)*

FIGURE 8.4. Dino windsurfing at age ten *(Photo courtesy of Pamela Karydas)*

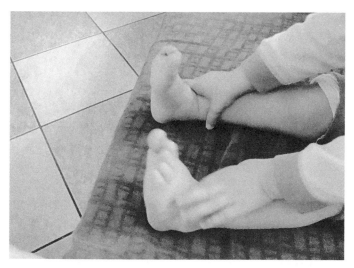

FIGURE 8.5. A beautiful pair of corrected feet *(Photo courtesy of Katerina Haviara)*

What Kids Have to Say about Clubfoot

Isaac (see Figure 8.6) and Asher (see Figure 8.7) are brothers. Both were born with distal arthrogryposis and clubfoot and were successfully treated for clubfoot with the Ponseti method. Because of the combination of clubfoot and distal AMC, their clubfoot treatment was more involved than usual, and they needed some surgery. Each offers advice to other children who could be in a similar situation.

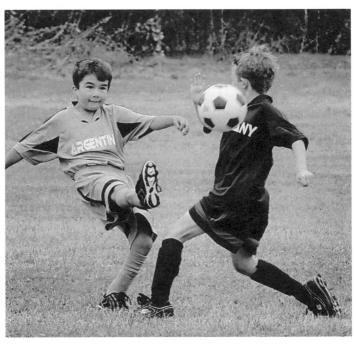

FIGURE 8.6. Isaac (left) playing soccer *(Photo courtesy of David Allen)*

Isaac's Advice (Age Eight)

It's sort of fun having casts because sometimes if you have surgery you can have a big, big surprise. Last time I had surgery, I got my DS.[1]

You could tell your parents what you want to have.

When you get your casts off, some people think the saw hurts, but it actually really tickles, and I actually like it myself. When you get it

[1] The Nintendo DS is a hand-held gaming console.

off, it's sort of weird because you haven't walked in a long time, and it's really hard to walk and run, but then it'll feel all better, and you can start to run and stuff.

When you get your stitches, it's just like being asleep. Your mind's just blank, and you don't hear or feel anything, and when you wake up you don't feel anything, and about two hours later, you don't remember anything before or after your surgery.

When you have a wheelchair, you'll get lots of attention, and you can go really fast but be careful. I'm the fifth-fastest person in the whole entire third grade at my school.

Asher's Advice (Age Six)

Hi, my name is Asher. If you're gonna go through lots of casts, ask your mom if you can have something special. Ask them really nicely. And they'll say "Yes" or "No."

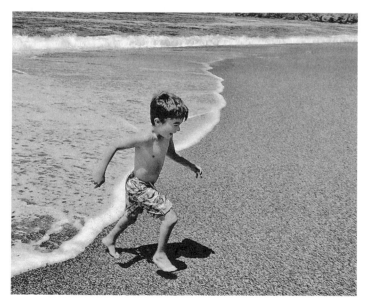

FIGURE 8.7. Asher running at the beach *(Photo courtesy of David Allen)*

If your cast feels really, really tight, you should always tell the person who's giving you the cast, and they'll take it off, and then they can pick another color and redo it, and you can just go home, and you can feel fine.

If you have lots of casts and your mom and dad really want you to wear tennis shoes and you like to wear flip flops a lot you should listen to them. And they might say, "Oh, I'm getting really worried." Because they don't want you to have any more casts, so you should wear your right shoes.

When you're in a wheelchair at school, some people might make fun of the wheelchair. However, the yard duty teacher will make you feel better.

When you have surgery, if you're gonna have it like when it's Christmas Eve, don't be worried that you won't get any presents because Santa will come and give you presents. If you stay overnight in the hospital, this is my favorite part—you get to eat in bed and watch lots of movies, and it's really fun. If you take dances like hip hop or like jazz that are sort of active, don't be worried about your kids because they can run and be active.

Straight, Strong, and Stretchy: A Children's Clubfoot Story

Ryan was born with a clubfoot. His parents took him to a clubfoot doctor when he was a little baby. The doctor stretched his foot for a

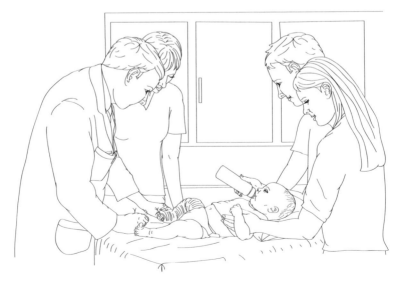

minute or two until it was straighter. Then he put a cast on Ryan's leg for a week to help his foot stay put.

Ryan's parents took him to the doctor every week. Each time, the doctor stretched his foot and put on a new cast. Finally the last cast came off. Ryan's foot was nice and straight, but that was not enough.

To keep his foot straight, Ryan wore a clubfoot brace. At first he wore his brace all the time. When Ryan was older, he wore his brace only at nighttime.

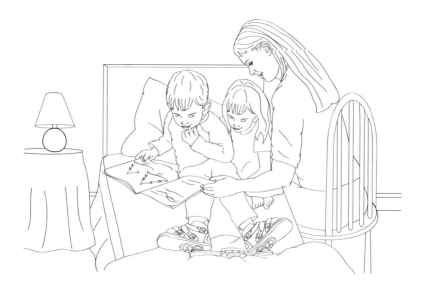

The brace kept Ryan's foot straight, but that was not enough. He needed strong legs and feet, too.

Ryan loved to play. He climbed the ladder at the playground and went down the slide. He chased his sister Anna and she chased him. He pedaled his tricycle with his friend Michael.

Playing helped Ryan's feet and legs grow strong, but that was not enough. They needed to be stretchy, too.

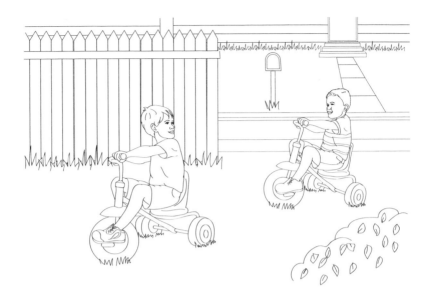

Ryan stretched like a runner before a race. Sometimes he played on a trampoline. Ryan bounced up and down, up and down. Bouncing on the trampoline helped Ryan's feet get strong and stay stretchy at the same time.

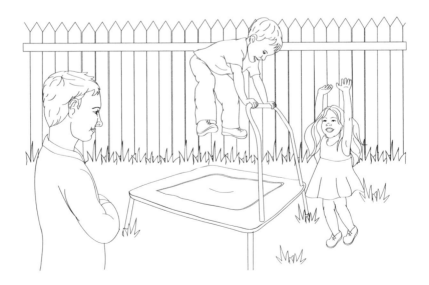

Even though he ran and played without a brace in the daytime, Ryan still wore a brace at night. After bath time and pajamas, Ryan put on his socks and smoothed them out so there were no wrinkles. Sometimes he needed a little help.

When his socks were just right, it was time to put on the first shoe. Ryan's shoes looked like sandals but they were specially made for his brace. Some children wear other kinds of special shoes with their clubfoot braces.

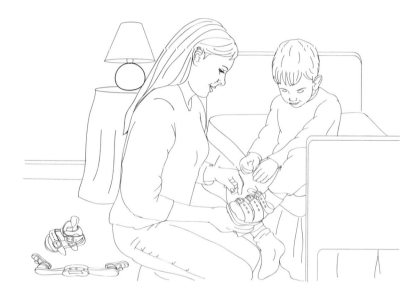

Ryan put on his shoe and stepped down so that his foot went all the way inside. Mom pulled the shoe straps nice and tight and buckled them. She checked to make sure she could see his heel and his toes.

Then, Ryan's sister Anna brought the bar. She loved to click the bar and always helped. Click, click! Anna helped snap the bar onto Ryan's shoes.

Ryan pretended his brace was a snowboard. Then he climbed into bed, cozy and warm. He would sleep all night wearing his brace.

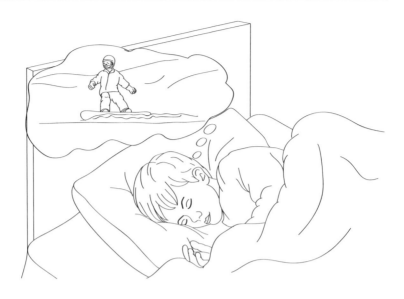

One day, when Ryan was five, his mom and dad took him to see the clubfoot doctor again. The doctor asked Ryan to take off his shoes and socks. He checked Ryan's foot while he was sitting down.

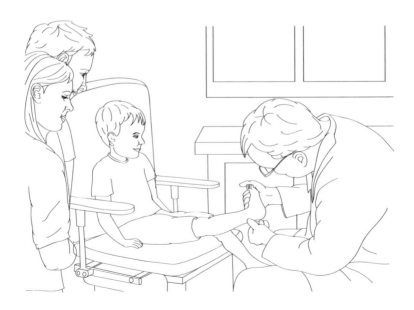

He checked Ryan's foot when he was standing up and walking around.

"That's enough," said the doctor. "You don't need to wear a brace anymore."

Ryan was glad his foot was straight. But then he thought about the fun he had keeping his feet and legs strong and stretchy. "Oh," said Ryan sadly.

"What's wrong?" asked his dad.

"Can I still stretch like a runner and play on the trampoline?" he asked.

"Of course," said Dad. And that's what Ryan did.

Appendix: Clubfoot Assessment

Doctors use a variety of assessment methods to determine how severe clubfoot is for individual children and to check how their feet improve during treatment. Typically, a doctor selects one method and uses it consistently in a systematic way, rather than using several different methods. This chapter describes the following methods:

- clubfoot severity scale (Diméglio scale)
- Pirani severity score
- Caroll score

During serial casting, you should be able to see that your child's foot looks better each time a cast is removed. As a parent, you do not need to know how to do the assessments.

Clubfoot Severity Scale (Diméglio Scale)

This scale is from 0 to 20, with a score of 0 representing a normal foot. Feet are divided into four groups:

0–5: normal feet or feet with mild symptoms that can be easily moved into a normal position

6–10: flexible feet that can move toward a more normal position

11–15: the feet are somewhat resistant, but not completely stiff

16–20: very severe clubfoot

The Diméglio Method of Scoring Clubfoot

Equinus	0	Dorsiflexion 20°+
	1	Dorsiflexion 0° to 20°
	2	Plantarflexion 0° to –20°
	3	Plantarflexion –20° to –45°
	4	Plantarflexion –45° to –90°
Varus	0	Valgus 20°+
	1	Valgus 0° to 20°
	2	Varus 0° to –20°
	3	Varus –20° to –45°
	4	Varus –45° to –90°
Supination	0	Pronation 20°+
	1	Pronation 0° to 20°
	2	Supination 0° to –20°
	3	Supination –20° to –45°
	4	Supination –45° to –90°
Adductus	0	Abduction 20°+
	1	Abduction 0° to 20°
	2	Adduction 0° to –20°
	3	Adduction –20° to –45°
	4	Adduction –45° to –90°
Posterior crease where the heel meets the ankle	0	No
	1	Yes
Medial crease on the sole of the foot	0	No
	1	Yes
Cavus	0	No
	1	Yes
Deviant muscle function	0	No
	1	Yes

Pirani Severity Score

This is used to assess an unoperated clubfoot for a child up to two years of age. This method uses six elements to rate the severity of the clubfoot. Each element is scored as 0 (normal), 0.5 (moderate), or 1 (severe). The scores are added up.

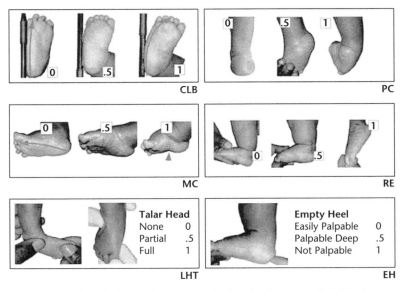

FIGURE 10.1. The Pirani severity score evaluates six elements of clubfoot. (Images are from the publication *Clubfoot: Ponseti Management*, 3rd ed., by Lynn Staheli, Ignacio Ponseti, et al., courtesy of Global HELP, http://www.global-help.org/publications/books/help_cfponseti.pdf.)

Caroll Score

The following table shows the criteria used to determine a Caroll score. A person's Caroll score is based on ten different problems that can occur with clubfoot.

The Criteria Used to Determine a Caroll Score

Caroll Score	Medical Name	Description
1	Calf atrophy	The calf muscle is weak. If only one foot is affected, this calf muscle is smaller than the other one.
2	Posterior fibula	The fibula is the smaller of two calf bones. Posterior means the back part of the leg.
3	Creases	Creases can be seen on the bottom of the foot or at the front of the ankle.
4	Curved lateral border	The side of the foot curves inward.
5	Cavus	The foot has a very high arch.
6	Navicular fixed to medial malleolus	The navicular bone, one of the tarsal bones in the foot, stays next to the ankle bone.
7	Calcaneus fixed to fibula	The heel bone does not move away from the fibula (calf bone).
8	Fixed equinus	The ankle has limited movement. The foot cannot flex upward as far as a normal foot would.
9	Fixed adductus	The foot bends toward the midline of the body and stays that way.
10	Fixed forefoot supination	The foot tilts sideways so the outside of the foot is toward the floor.

Glossary

abduction. Moving a limb outward away from the center, or midline, of the body.

adduction. Moving a limb inward toward the midline of the body.

Achilles tendon. Also called the heel cord, this tendon is located in the back of the ankle. It connects the calf muscle to the heel.

Achilles tenotomy. Surgery in which the doctor cuts the Achilles tendon to allow the heel to drop downward. The tendon will regrow.

AFO (ankle–foot orthosis). A foot brace that can be used together with a foot abduction brace (FAB) to treat clubfoot. An AFO alone cannot effectively treat clubfoot.

anesthesiologist. A doctor who completed an internship and residency in anesthesiology and is certified by the American Board of Anesthesiologists.

anterior. In the front or from the front.

anterior tibialis tendon transfer (ATTT). Surgery in which this tendon is transferred to a different location in the foot to keep clubfoot from coming back.

arthrogryposis. A rare congenital disorder that causes multiple joint contractures.

atypical clubfoot. Also called complex clubfoot, this type of clubfoot is more severe than usual. The foot can be short and stubby. There is a crease on the sole of the foot and in some cases there is also a crease at the top of the heel.

bilateral. Affecting both sides.

calcaneus. Also called the calcis, this is the heelbone.

clubfoot. A disorder in which the foot is turned downward and inward at birth and remains in this position.

collagen. A strong, fibrous protein in connective tissues and bones.

congenital. Present at birth.

deformed. The wrong shape.

Denis Browne brace. A brace that is used to treat clubfoot.

dorsal. Located on the top side.

dorsiflexion. The foot's ability to flex upward.

epidural. Pain medicine that is given through a soft tube called a catheter into the epidural space, which is near the backbone and spinal cord.

equinovarus. A medical term that means clubfoot.

eversion. The foot is turned or rotated outward.

FAB (foot abduction brace). A brace used to maintain clubfoot correction after serial casting.

French method. A method of correcting clubfoot in which physical therapy and taping are used instead of stretching and casts.

geneticist. A doctor who has studied genetics and is certified by the American Board of Medical Genetics.

heel-cord tenotomy. See Achilles tenotomy.

hydrocolloidal bandage. A special kind of bandage made for open sores or burns.

hypotonia. Low muscle tone.

idiopathic. Occurring spontaneously or with an unknown cause.

incentive spirometer. A device used to encourage a patient to breathe deeply after surgery.

incision. The cut a doctor makes in order to do surgery.

inversion. The foot is rotated or turned inward.

ligaments. Bands of tough tissue that connect bones together.

low muscle tone. Poor muscle tone; less strength than usual.

maceration. A complication affecting the skin that can occur if the skin gets wet inside the cast.

manipulation. Adjusting the position of the foot to bring it into better alignment.

neuromuscular clubfoot. Clubfoot associated with neuromuscular problems or nerve damage.

nonsteroidal anti-inflammatory drug (NSAID). These drugs offer pain relief and reduce inflammation. Some common examples are ibuprofen and aspirin.

orthopedist. A doctor who treats problems with muscles and bones. Also see pediatric orthopedic surgeon.

orthotist. An orthotist makes and fits orthopedic harnesses and braces prescribed by doctors.

ossification. The process of cartilage hardening into bone. This is a normal development in babies.

osteoarthritis. A joint disease in which the cartilage wears away or breaks down, causing pain and inflammation.

patient-controlled anesthesia (PCA). Pain medication in a pump that is controlled by a patient, who pushes a button as needed to get more pain medicine.

pediatric orthopedic surgeon. A doctor who treats problems with muscles and bones in babies and children.

pediatrician. A doctor who specializes in treating children.

percutaneous. Through the skin. For a percutaneous tenotomy, the doctor "pokes" a very small scalpel through the skin as if using a needle.

physical therapist. A physical therapist is trained to work with people of all ages to prevent the onset, or reduce the progression, of conditions resulting from disease, injury, or other causes.

plantigrade. When standing, the sole of the foot is flat on the floor in a normal position.

plantar surface. The bottom of the foot.

plastizote. A foam rubber–type padding used to prevent blisters in shoes or AFOs.

podiatrist. A podiatrist (doctor of podiatric medicine) specializes in diagnosing, treating, and preventing foot problems.

Ponseti method. A method of treating clubfoot that uses gentle stretching and a series of casts to correct the foot, followed by brace wear.

positional clubfoot. The foot has the appearance of a clubfoot, but it is flexible and can easily move into normal alignment. This is caused by the position of the baby's foot before birth. Many doctors do not consider this to be true clubfoot.

pressure sore. A wound caused by pressure against the skin for a prolonged period of time.

prostaglandins. Hormones that produce inflammation and pain.

relapse. The return of symptoms or a medical problem after there has been improvement.

remodeling. An ongoing normal process in which new bone gradually grows, and old bone tissue is absorbed.

risk factors. Reasons why a person is more likely to have a medical condition.

scoliosis. A condition in which the spine is curved.

serial casting. A series of casts applied one after another after each Ponseti treatment to hold the clubfoot in a straighter position.

spina bifida. A birth defect affecting the spinal cord that involves the neural tube.

talipes equinovarus (TEV). A medical term that means clubfoot.

tenotomy. Surgery in which the doctor makes a small cut to allow a tendon to grow longer.

tendons. The connective tissues that attach muscles to bones.

tibia. The shinbone. It is one of two bones between the knee and the ankle.

unilateral. Affecting one side.

valgus. Turned outward away from the midline of the body.

varus. Turned inward toward the midline of the body.

X ray. A form of electromagnetic radiation. In a health-care setting, a machine sends X rays through the body. A computer or special film records the images that are created.

Bibliography

Internet Sources

American Academy of Pediatrics. "What Is a Pediatric Geneticist?" 2002. http://www.healthychildren.org/English/family-life/health -management/pediatric-specialists/Pages/What-is-a-Pediatric -Geneticist.aspx (accessed 25 October 2011).

American Academy of Pediatrics. "What Is a Pediatric Orthopedic Surgeon?" 2000. http://www.healthychildren.org/English/family-life /health-management/pediatric-specialists/Pages/What-is-a-Pedi atric-Orthopedic-Surgeon.aspx (accessed 25 October 2011).

American College of Radiology (ACR) and the Radiological Society of North America (RSNA), "Radiation Exposure in X-ray Examinations." 2005. http://www.radiologyinfo.org.

Chen, H. "Arthrogryposis." http://www.emedicine.com/ped/TOPIC142 .HTM (accessed 19 October 2011).

Children's Hospital Boston. "Clubfoot." 2010. http://www.childrens hospital.org/az/Site1159/mainpageS1159P0.html (accessed 19 October 2011).

Children's Memorial Hospital, Pediatric Specialties. "Fetal Clubfoot." http://www.childrensmemorial.org/depts/fetalhealth/clubfoot.aspx (accessed 19 October 2011).

MedlinePlus, The Patient Education Institute, Inc. "Clubfoot Overview." Updated 28 April 2011. http://www.nlm.nih.gov/medlineplus /tutorials/clubfootoverview/htm/_no_50_no_0.htm.

Ponseti International Website for Parents. "How to Recognize the Ponseti Method." http://ponseti.info/parents/index.php?option=com _content&task=view&id=57&Itemid=67 (accessed 19 October 2011).

Ponseti International Website for Parents, "Relapses and Bracing for

Children Treated with the Ponseti Method." http://ponseti.info
/parents/index.php?option=com_content&task=view&id=25&
Itemid=40 (accessed 19 October 2011).

Schroeder, S., E. Sella, P. Blume, and R. O'Hara. "Triple Arthrodesis."
2008. http://emedicine.medscape.com/article/1234042-overview
(accessed 19 October 2011).

Ponseti, I. "Commonly Asked Questions on Clubfoot Treatment."
http://ponseti.info/parents/index.php?option=com_content&task
=view&id=40&Itemid=61 (accessed 19 October 2011).

University of California San Francisco. "Learn More: Amniotic Band
Syndrome." 2008. http://fetus.ucsfmedicalcenter.org/amniotic/learn
_more.asp (accessed 19 October 2011).

Wheeless, C. R. "Talipes Equinovarus/Clubfoot." In *Wheeless' Textbook of Orthopaedics*. Durham, NC: Duke Orthopedics, 1996–2005.
http://www.wheelessonline.com/ortho/talipes_equinovarus_club
foot (accessed 19 October 2011).

Wheeless, C. R. *Wheeless' Textbook of Orthopaedics.*
"Myelomeningocele Clubfoot." In *Wheeless' Textbook of Orthopaedics*. Durham, NC: Duke Orthopedics, 1996–2005. http://www.whee
lessonline.com/ortho/myelomeningocele_club_foot (accessed 19
October 2011).

Books and Booklets

Ponseti, I. *Congenital Clubfoot: Fundamentals of Treatment*. New York:
Oxford University Press, 1996.

Quamat, "Infant Massage Strokes, Legs." http://quamut.com/quamut
/infant_massage/page/infant_massage_strokes.html.

Staheli, L., I. Ponseti, and Others. *Clubfoot: Ponseti Management*.
3rd ed. Seattle, WA: Global HELP, 2009.

Wood, W., R. B. Lovell, and R. T. Winter. "The Foot, Assessment of
Clubfoot by Severity Scale." In *Lovell and Winter's Pediatric Orthopaedics*. 6th ed., ed. R. T. Morrissey and S. L. Weinstein. Philadel-
phia, PA: Lippincott Williams & Wilkins, 2005. 1266.

Wood, W., R. B. Lovell, and R. T. Winter. "The French, or Functional,
Method of Treatment for Clubfoot," In *Lovell and Winter's Pediatric
Orthopaedics*. 6th ed., ed. R. T. Morrissey and S. L. Weinstein. New
York: Lippincott Williams & Wilkins, 2005. 1270.

Journal Articles

Chen, R. C., J. E. Gordan, S. J. Luhmann, P. L. Schoenecker, and M. B. Dobbs. "A New Dynamic Foot Abduction Orthosis for Clubfoot Treatment." *Journal of Pediatric Orthopedics* 27 (2007): 522–28.

Colburn, M., and M. Williams. "Evaluation of the Treatment of Idiopathic Clubfoot by Using the Ponseti Method." *Journal of Foot and Ankle Surgery* 42, no. 5 (2003): 259–67. http://www.ncbi.nlm.nih .gov/pubmed/14566717 (accessed 19 October 2011).

Dobbs, M. B., and C. A. Gurnett. "Update on Clubfoot: Etiology and Treatment." *Clinical Orthopaedics and Related Research* 467, no. 5 (2009): 1146–53. http://www.ncbi.nlm.nih.gov/pubmed/19224303 (accessed 19 October 2011).

Dobbs, M. B., D. Purcell, R. Nunley, and J. Morcuende. "Early Results of a New Method of Treatment for Idiopathic Congenital Vertical Talus." *Journal of Bone and Joint Surgery* 89-A, Suppl. 2, Pt. 1 (2007): 111–21. http://www.ncbi.nlm.nih.gov/pubmed/17332130 (accessed 19 October 2011).

Dobbs, M. B., J. R. Rudzki, D. B. Purcell, T. Walton, K. R. Porter, and C. A. Gurnett. "Factors Predictive of Outcome After Use of the Ponseti Method for the Treatment of Idiopathic Clubfeet." *Journal of Bone and Joint Surgery, Am* 86 (2004): 22–27. http://www.jbjs.org /article.aspx?articleid=26188 (accessed 19 October 2011).

Glotzbecker, M. P., J. A. Estroff, S. A. Spencer, J. C. Bosley, R. B. Parad, J. R. Kasser, and S. T. Mahan. "Prenatally Diagnosed Clubfeet: Comparing Ultrasonographic Severity with Objective Clinical Outcomes." *Journal of Pediatric Orthopedics* 30, no. 6 (2010): 606–11. http://www.ncbi.nlm.nih.gov/pubmed/20733428.

Gurnett, C. A., F. Alaee, L. M. Kruse, D. M. Desruisseau, J. T. Hecht, C. A. Wise, A. M. Bowcock, and M. B. Dobbs. "Asymmetric Lower-Limb Malformations in Individuals with Homeobox PITX1 Gene Mutation." *American Journal of Human Genetics* 83, no. 5 (2008): 616–22. http://www.ncbi.nlm.nih.gov/pubmed/18950742 (accessed 20 October 2011).

Janicki, J. A., U. G. Narayanan, B. J. Harvey, A. Roy, S. Weir, and J. G. Wright. "Comparison of Surgeon and Physiotherapist-Directed Ponseti Treatment of Idiopathic Clubfoot." *The Journal of Bone and*

Joint Surgery, Am 91 (2009): 1101–1108. http://www.ncbi.nlm.nih.gov /pubmed/19411458 (accessed 19 October 2011).

Kalenderer, O., A. Reisoglu, A. Turgut, and H. Agus. "Evaluation of Clinical and Radiographic Outcomes of Complete Subtalar Release in Clubfoot Treatment." *Journal of the American Podiatric Medical Association* 98, (no. 6 (2008): 451–56. http://www.ncbi.nlm.nih.gov /pubmed/19017853 (accessed 19 October 2011).

Karol, L. A., K. Jeans, and R. ElHawary. "Gait Analysis after Initial Non-operative Treatment for Clubfeet: Intermediate Term Followup at Age 5, Symposium: Clubfoot: Etiology and Treatment," *Clinical Orthopaedics and Related Research* 467, no. 5 (2009): 1206–1213. http:// www.clinorthop.org/journal/11999/167/5/702_10.1007_ä11999-008 -0702-9/2008/Gait_Analysis_after_Initial_Nonoperative_Treat ment.html (accessed 19 October 2011).

Lourenço, A. F., and J. A. Morcuende. "Correction of Neglected Idio-pathic Club Foot by the Ponseti Method." *Journal of Bone and Joint Surgery, Br* 89-B, no. 3 (2007): 378–81. http://www.ncbi.nlm.nih.gov /pubmed/17356154 (accessed 19 October 2011).

Mitchell, P. D., M. Tisdall, and H. G. Zadeh. "Selective Botulinum Toxin Injection in the Treatment of Recurrent Deformity Following Surgi-cal Correction of Club Foot: A Preliminary Report of 3 Children." *Acta Orthopaedica Scandinavica* 75, no. 5 (2004): 630–33. http:// www.ncbi.nlm.nih.gov/pubmed/15513498 (accessed 19 October 2011).

Morcuende, J. A., L. A. Dolan, F. R. Dietz, and I. V. Ponseti. "Radical Reduction in the Rate of Extensive Corrective Surgery for Club-foot Using the Ponseti Method." *Pediatrics* 113, no. 2 (2004): 376–80. http://www.ncbi.nlm.nih.gov/pubmed?term=14754952 (accessed 19 October 2011).

Morcuende, J. A., and M. G. Vitale. "Non-invasive Method Is Gold Standard for Treating Clubfoot." *AAP News* 27 (2006): 18. http://aap news.aappublications.org/content/27/9/18.2.citation (accessed 19 October 2011).

Ponseti, I., M. Zhivkov, N. Davis, M. Sinclair, M. B. Dobbs, and J. A. Morcuende. "Treatment of the Complex Idiopathic Clubfoot." *Clini-cal Orthopaedics and Related Research* 451 (2006): 171–6, http://www .ncbi.nlm.nih.gov/pubmed/16788408 (accessed 19 October 2011).

Richards, B., S. Faulks, K. E. Rathjen, L. A. Karol, C. E. Johnston, and S. A. Jones. "A Comparison of Two Nonoperative Methods of Idiopathic Clubfoot Correction: The Ponseti Method and the French Functional (Physiotherapy) Method." *Journal of Bone and Joint Surgery, Am* 90, no. 11 (2008): 2313–21. http://www.ncbi.nlm.nih.gov/pubmed/18978399 (accessed 19 October 2011).

van Bosse, H. J., S. Marangoz, W. B. Lehman, and D. A. Sala. "Correction of Arthrogrypotic Clubfoot with a Modified Ponseti Technique, Symposium: Clubfoot: Etiology and Treatment." *Clinical Orthopaedics and Related Research* 467, no. 5 (2009): 1283–93. http://www.springerlink.com/content/d78t252l77750471 (accessed 19 October 2011).

Wainwright, A. M., T. Auld, M. K. Benson, and T. N. Theologis. "The Classification of Congenital Talipes Equinovarus." *Journal of Bone and Joint Surgery, Br* 84B, no. 7 (2002): 1020–24. http://www.ncbi.nlm.nih.gov/pubmed/12358365 (accessed 19 October 2011).

Resources

This chapter provides additional resources pertaining to clubfoot and children's health.

Clubfoot Information and Support Groups

Though every effort has been made to select online content that is likely to remain available, the information on websites and their location can change. If you have trouble locating a resource, try a search. Searching is also a good way to discover new information that may have been put online after this list was created.

A Different Foot is a website with information about complex clubfoot, also called atypical clubfoot.
http://adifferentfoot.freeservers.com/index.html

Amelia's Journey is a blog about a child's ATTT surgery for clubfoot treatment.
http://journey2amelia.blogspot.com/2008/10/attt-surgery.html

AMC Support provides support and information about arthrogryposis multiplex congenita (AMC).
www.amcsupport.org

Clubfoot Club is a website created by a parent of a child with clubfoot. It is set up to accept donated clubfoot orthotics and to allow people to sponsor clubfoot treatment in the developing world.
www.clubfootclub.org

Clubfoot (Talipes equinovarus) physiotherapy by images. This website has photos of the French method of physical therapy for clubfoot.
http://clubfootfrance.free.fr/postures.htm

Congenital Clubfoot (Talipes) is a South African website about the Ponseti method of clubfoot treatment.
www.clubfoot.co.za

Global HELP provides low-cost or free health-education materials, such as "Clubfoot Guide for Parents," which is available in many languages.
www.global-help.org

MD Orthopaedics, Inc., produces and sells Ponseti clubfoot braces and Mitchell shoes.
(877) 766-7384 (877-Ponseti)
www.mdorthopaedics.com (or www.c-prodirect.co.uk in the UK)

Nosurgery4clubfoot is an online clubfoot support group.
http://health.groups.yahoo.com/group/nosurgery4clubfoot

One Perfect Pair, LLC, is an online shoe retailer for children with different-size feet.
(616) 425-8915
www.oneperfectpair.com

Our Journey to Lia is a blog that tells the story of Lia's adoption and treatment for clubfoot and hip dysplasia.
www.myadoptionwebsite.com/liashu/werehome040609.htm

Ponseti Clubfoot Center and Ponseti International Association (PIA) are affiliated with the University of Iowa, Department of Orthopaedics & Rehabilitation.
(319) 467-5107
www.ponseti.info/v1

STEPS Charity Worldwide (United Kingdom)
Telephone: +44 (0)1925 750271
www.steps-charity.org.uk/home.php

Where Will This Little Foot Take Him? is a mother's blog about her child's neuromuscular atypical clubfoot.
http://wherewillthislittlefoottakehim.blogspot.com

Foreign Language Resources

For clubfoot resources in many languages, see the listing for Global HELP at www.global-help.org.

Many Medline topics are available in other languages at www.nlm.nih.gov.

The topic "Information for Parents of Children with Clubfoot" is in Spanish and German at the website www.uihealthcare.com.

Socks, Shoes, and Sleep Sacks

The following were recommended by parents as good sources. For socks, you can try Baby Hanes brand socks, or SmartKnit AFO Socks. Some websites that carry them are:

AFO Socks
www.afosocks.com

Knit-Rite, Inc.
www.knitrite.com/orthotic-afo-spinal-interfaces.html.

For shoes that are generally comfortable for children with clubfeet, try See Kai Run shoes at the website www.seekairun.com or at Nordstrom department stores. Robeez shoes and New Balance shoes also work well for many children. For children who wear different-sized shoes, Nordstrom department stores allow you to buy a pair of shoes in two different sizes. There are several online retailers who sell different-sized shoes:

Healthy Shoe Store
www.healthyshoestore.com/conditions-different-sized-feet.html

Mixmatch Shoes
www.mixmatchshoes.com

One Perfect Pair
www.oneperfectpair.com

Odd Shoe Finder
www.oddshoefinder.com

For sleep sacks, try:
HALO SleepSack
www.halosleep.com (Also available at Target department stores.)

Financial Assistance

Air Care Alliance includes a number of nonprofit and charitable organizations that provide free or reduced-cost air transportation for patients in the United States.
(888) 260-9707
www.aircareall.org

Angel Flight, Inc., a member of Air Care Alliance, provides free air transportation to patients and their families, mainly to and from the Midwest including Iowa.
(918) 749-8992
www.angelflight.com

Children's Special Health Services (CSHS) offers assistance to families with special health-care needs. Services are available in each state in the United States through their health departments, though the names vary. For example, in North Dakota, see CSHS at www.ndhealth.gov/CSHS, and in California, see California Children's Services at www.dhcs.ca.gov/services/ccs/Pages/default.aspx.

Early Intervention Program for Infants and Toddlers with Disabilities is available in each state. This website gives an overview: www.ed.gov/programs/osepeip/index.html

Kya's Krusade provides resources for families affected by arthrogryposis, clubfoot, cerebral palsy, and other medical conditions.
(614) 750-2198
www.kyaskrusade.org

Miracle Feet is a nonprofit organization that helps deliver the Ponseti method of clubfoot treatment worldwide.
www.miraclefeet.org.

National Patient Travel Center helps patients in need of transportation for medical care.
(757) 512-5287; for patients: (800) 296-1217
www.patienttravel.org

Shriners Hospitals for Children treat children regardless of the family's ability to pay and can assist in transportation of patients to their facilities. Some of the hospitals have stronger clubfoot departments than others.
(800) 237-5055
www.shrinershq.org

Texas Scottish Rite Hospital for Children has a clubfoot treatment center that offers both the Ponseti method and a French physical therapy program. They provide healthcare to children residing in Texas regardless of the family's ability to pay.
(800) 421-1121   (214) 559-5000
www.tsrhc.org

Health and Medical Articles and Fact Sheets

This section lists articles relevant to clubfoot that are written for patients.

Agency for Healthcare Research and Quality (AHRQ), U.S. Department of Health and Human Services. "20 Tips to Help Prevent Medical Errors in Children." AHRQ Publication No. 02-P034, September 2002. http://archive.ahrq.gov/consumer/20tipkid.htm (accessed 18 October 2011).

American Society of Anesthesiologists. "When Your Child Needs Anesthesia." http://asatest.asahq.org/patientEducation/WhenYourChild NeedsAnesthesia.pdf (accessed 18 October 2011).

Children's Specialists of San Diego. "Ponseti Cast Care Instructions, Home Care Instructions for Clubfoot Casting." http://childrensspecial ists.com/body.cfm?id=507 (accessed 18 October 2011).

Connecticut Children's Medical Center. "Clubfoot." http://www.con necticutchildrens.org/body_dept.cfm?id=889 (accessed 18 October 2011).

Johns Hopkins Medicine. "Patient Guide to Clubfoot." http://www .hopkinsortho.org/clubfoot.html (accessed 25 October 2011).

Miller, Beth. "First Gene for Clubfoot Identified at Washington University School of Medicine." http://mednews.wustl.edu/news/page/normal /12803.html (accessed 18 October 2011).

Morcuende, Jose, interview by Dr. Mike from Pediacast. At www.pon seti.info, select Info for Parents > Video, and scroll down to click the link and listen to the podcast.

Mosca, Vincent S. "Clubfoot Guide for Parents." 2010. http://www .global-help.org/publications/books/book_cfparents.html (accessed 18 October 2011).

OrthoPediatrics Corp. "A Patient's Guide to Clubfoot." This guide includes diagrams of clubfoot surgery. http://www.orthopediatrics.com /docs/guides/clubfoot.html (accessed 18 October 2011).

Ponseti, Ignacio. "Commonly Asked Questions on Clubfoot Treatment." http://www.uihealthcare.com/topics/medicaldepartments /orthopaedics/clubfeet/questions.html (accessed 19 October 2011).

Ponseti, Ignacio. "To Parents of Children Born with Clubfeet." http://www.uihealthcare.com/topics/medicaldepartments/orthopaedics/clubfeet/parents.html (accessed 19 October 2011).

Ponseti International Association. "Relapses and Bracing for Children Treated with the Ponseti Method." http://ponseti.info/parents/index.php?option=com_content&task=view&id=25&Itemid=40 (accessed 18 October 2011).

Science News. "New Dynamic Brace Developed To Advance Clubfoot Treatment." ScienceDaily (5 July 2007). http://www.sciencedaily.com/releases/2007/06/070628161441.htm (accessed 18 October 2011).

Scottish Rite Hospital for Children. "French Functional (Physical Therapy) Method." http://www.tsrhc.org/french-functional-method.htm (accessed 18 October 2011).

SMARxT Disposal. "Throw Away Your Old Medicines Safely." http://www.ismp.org/consumers/throwAwayMedsSafely.asp (accessed 18 October 2011).

STEPS Charity, Case Histories. "Case Histories from Parents Whose Babies Were Diagnosed with Clubfoot During an Ultrasound Scan." http://www.steps-charity.org.uk/links/8-87-prenatal_diagnosis.php (accessed 18 October 2011).

UCL Institute of Child Health. "Looking after Your Child's Ankle Foot Orthosis (AFO) Information for Families." http://www.gosh.nhs.uk/gosh_families/information_sheets/orthosis_ankle_foot/orthosis_ankle_foot_discharge.html (accessed 25 October 2011).

Your Orthopaedic Connection. "Clubfoot." http://orthoinfo.aaos.org/topic.cfm?topic=A00255 (accessed 18 October 2011).

Health and Medical Organizations

These organizations provide educational health and medical information or medical equipment. They cannot give medical advice or answer questions about an individual's condition. Contact your doctor with specific questions about your child's personal medical treatment.

American Academy of Pediatrics (AAOP)
(847) 434-4000
www.aap.org

American Board of Medical Genetics
(301) 634-7315
http://genetics.faseb.org/genetics/abmg.html

American Board of Pediatrics
(919) 929-0461
E-mail: abpeds@abpeds.org

Automotive Safety Program, Special Needs Transportation
(800) 543-6227   (317) 944-2977
www.preventinjury.org

Avenues (arthrogryposis support)
(209) 928-3688
www.avenuesforamc.com

Centers for Medicare & Medicaid Services (CMS)
Also administers State Children's Health Insurance (SCHIP), Health
Insurance Portability and Accountability Act (HIPAA)
(800) 267-2323   (410) 786-3000
www.cms.hhs.gov

Easter Seals
(800) 221-6827   (312) 726-6200
www.easterseals.com

Healthfinder, National Health Information Center, U.S. Department of
Health and Human Services at www.healthfinder.gov

March of Dimes Foundation
(914) 997-4488
www.marchofdimes.com

MedlinePlus, Medical encyclopedia, dictionary, and health topics in
many languages at www.nlm.nih.gov

National Institutes of Health
(301) 496-4000   TTY: (301) 402-9612
www.nih.gov; for publications: http://catalog.niams.nih.gov

Pediatric Orthopaedic Society of North America (POSNA)
(847) 698-1692
www.posna.org

PubMed, a free digital archive service of the National Library of Medicine
www.pubmed.gov

Medical Publications

The documents listed in this section were written for medical professionals such as doctors and nurses. They are presented here for those readers who are comfortable with medical and scientific terminology. The listings are formatted in a style that makes it easy to locate them in medical databases such as PubMed. For more medical publications, see the Bibliography.

Alvarado, D. M., H. Aferol, K. McCall, J. B. Huang, M. Techy, J. Buchan, J. Cady, P. R. Gonzales, M. B. Dobbs, and C. A. Gurnett. "Familial Isolated Clubfoot Is Associated with Recurrent Chromosome 17q23.1q23.2 Microduplications Containing TBX4." *American Journal of Human Genetics* 87, no. 1 (2010): 154–60. http://www.ncbi.nlm.nih.gov/pmc/articles/PMC2896772 (accessed 19 October 2011).

Chu, A., A. S. Labar, D. A. Sala, H. J. van Bosse, and W. B. Lehman. "Clubfoot Classification: Correlation with Ponseti Cast Treatment." *Journal of Pediatric Orthopedics* 30, no. 7 (2010): 695–99. http://www.ncbi.nlm.nih.gov/pubmed/20864855 (accessed 19 October 2011).

Dobbs, M. B., J. A. Morcuende, C. A. Gurnett, and I. V. Ponseti. "Treatment of Idiopathic Clubfoot: An Historical Review." *Iowa Orthopaedic Journal* 20 (2000): 59–64. http://www.ncbi.nlm.nih.gov/pubmed/10934626 (accessed 19 October 2011).

Gerlach, D. J., C. A. Gurnett, N. Limpaphayom, F. Alaee, Z. Zhang, K. Porter, M. Kirchhofer, M. D. Smyth, and M. B. Dobbs. "Early Results of the Ponseti Method for the Treatment of Clubfoot Associated with Myelomeningocele." *Journal of Bone and Joint Surgery, Am* 91, no. 6 (2009): 1350–9. http://www.ncbi.nlm.nih.gov/pubmed/19487512 (accessed 19 October 2011).

Gottschalk, H. P., L. A. Karol, and K. A. Jeans. "Gait Analysis of Children Treated for Moderate Clubfoot with Physical Therapy Versus the Ponseti Cast Technique." *Journal of Pediatric Orthopedics* 30, no. 3 (2010): 235–39. http://www.ncbi.nlm.nih.gov/pubmed/20357588 (accessed 19 October 2011).

Iltar, S., M. Uysal, K. B. Alemdaroglu, N. H. Aydogan, T. Kara, and D. Atlihan. "Treatment of Clubfoot with the Ponseti Method: Should We Begin Casting in the Newborn Period or Later? *Journal of Foot and Ankle Surgery* 49, no. 5 (2010): 426–31. http://www.ncbi.nlm.nih.gov/pubmed/20797585 (accessed 19 October 2011).

Ng, B. K., T. P. Lam, and J. C. Cheng. "Treatment of Severe Clubfoot with Manipulation Using Synthetic Cast Material and a Foam-casting Platform: A Preliminary Report." *Journal of Pediatric Orthopaedics*, Part B 19, no. 2 (2010): 164–70. http://www.ncbi.nlm.nih.gov/pubmed /19918191 (accessed 19 October 2011).

Nilgün, B., E. Suat, S. I. Engin, U. Fatma, and Y. Yakut. "Short-term Results of Intensive Physiotherapy in Clubfoot Deformity Treated with Ponseti Method." *Pediatrics International* 53, no. 3 (2010): 381–85. http://www.ncbi.nlm.nih.gov/pubmed/20831648 (accessed 19 October 2011).

Noonan, K. J., and B. S. Richards. "Nonsurgical Management of Idiopathic Clubfoot." *Journal of the American Academy of Orthopaedic Surgeons* 11, no. 6 (2003): 392–402. http://www.ncbi.nlm.nih.gov/pubmed /14686824 (accessed 19 October 2011).

Ponseti, I. V., M. Zhivkov, N. Davis, M. Sinclair, M. B. Dobbs, and J. A. Morcuende. "Treatment of the Complex Idiopathic Clubfoot." *Clinical Orthopaedics and Related Research* 451 (2006): 171–6. http://www.ncbi .nlm.nih.gov/pubmed/16788408 (accessed 19 October 2011).

Steinman, S., B. S. Richards, S. Faulks, and K. Kaipus. "A Comparison of Two Nonoperative Methods of Idiopathic Clubfoot Correction: The Ponseti Method and the French Functional (Physiotherapy) Method." *Journal of Bone and Joint Surgery, Am* 91, Suppl 2 (2009): 299–312. http://www.ncbi.nlm.nih.gov/pubmed/19805592 (accessed 19 October 2011).

van Gelder, J. H., A. G. van Ruiten, J. D. Visser, and P. G. Maathuis. "Long-term Results of the Posteromedial Release in the Treatment of Idiopathic Clubfoot." *Journal of Pediatric Orthopedics* 30, no. 7 (2010): 700–704. http://www.ncbi.nlm.nih.gov/pubmed/20864856 (accessed 19 October 2011).

Zionts, L. E., and F. R. Dietz. "Bracing Following Correction of Idiopathic Clubfoot Using the Ponseti Method." *Journal of the American Academy of Orthopaedic Surgeons* 18, no. 8 (2010): 486–93. http://www .ncbi.nlm.nih.gov/pubmed/20675641 (accessed 19 October 2011).

Physician Education

POSNA Physician Education. "Infant Clubfoot." http://www.posna.org /education/StudyGuide/clubfootInfant.asp (accessed 19 October 2011).

Index

Italicized page references indicate figure illustrations. Tables are indicated with "t" following the page number.

Mitchell pressure saddles, 71, *71*, 80
Mitchell shoes: brace-fitting tips, 74,
    75, 87; description and overview,
    68, 70, *70*; skin problems with,
    79–80
mobility limitations, 5
mole foam/moleskin, 52, 80–81
Morcuende, Jose, 66–67, 92, 93
Motrin, 57, 76
movement, 56, 75, 76
muscle development and strength, 3,
    36, 90, 108, 125. *See also* hypotonia
muscle spasms, 108

N
naproxen (Naprosyn), 57
National Patient Travel Center, 26
navicular bones, 3, *3*
neoprene, 88
nerve problems, 4, 5, 23–24, 42, 48,
    106
Norco, 108
nosurgery4clubfoot, 12, 31
nurse practitioners, 24–25

O
orthotists, 25, 73–74
ossification, 20
overcorrection, 41, 45
oxycodone (Oxydose), 109

P
pain and pain management: arthritis,
    111; and braces, 76, 81; and casts,
    52, 56–57; muscle strengthening,
    44; overview, 56; postcasting, 56;
    relapse corrections, 44; surgery, 17,
    38, 39, 101–102; surgery recovery
    and, 39, 107, 108–109; with un-
    treated clubfoot, 5; walking and, 17
parents: brace experiences, 55, 77, 80,

87, 88; casting and recasting ex-
    periences, 43–44, 49; coping with
    casting, 58; coping with diagnoses,
    7–9; coping with treatments, 16–17;
    correction news and experiences,
    89; doctor-selection experiences,
    13, 14; postcasting experiences, 50;
    relapse experiences, 48; shoe tips,
    45; sibling experiences, 61–63; sur-
    gery experiences, 40, 49, 104–105;
    treatment experiences, 2, 8, 9, 16
parking permits for temporary dis-
    abilities, 49, 59
PAs. *See* physician's assistants
patient-controlled anesthesia (PCA),
    107
Pavlik harnesses, 23
pediatricians, 25
Pediatric Orthopedic Society of
    North America (POSNA), 1, 11
people reactions, 59
physical examinations, 6–7, 67
physical therapists (PTs), 25
physical therapy: early interven-
    tion services for, 95; for flexi-
    bility and strength building, 45,
    95–96; French, as clubfoot treat-
    ment method, 10, 97; health-care
    workers of, 25; as relapse treat-
    ment, 41
physician's assistants (PAs), 25
PIA. *See* Ponseti International As-
    sociation
Pirani severity score, 7, 122, 124, *124*
plantarflexion, 18, *19*
plantarflexion stops, 72
plantarflexion stop sandals, 72
plantigrade, 18, 19, 20
plastizote, 81
playing, 90–91
PMR (posteromedial release), 110